How to Fight AGEING

AF624052

How to Fight AGEING

Parvesh Handa

PEACOCK BOOKS

Published by
PEACOCK BOOKS
7/22, Ansari Road, Darya Ganj,
New Delhi-110002
Phones : +91-11-40775252, 23273880, 23275880, 23280451
Fax : +91-11-23285873
Web : www.atlanticbooks.com
E-mail : orders@atlanticbooks.com

Branch Office
5, Nallathambi Street, Wallajah Road,
Chennai-600002
Phones : +91-44-64611085, 32413319
E-mail : chennai@atlanticbooks.com

Peacock Books is an imprint of
Atlantic Publishers and Distributors (P) Ltd

Copyright © The Author, 2010

All rights reserved. No part of this publication may be reproduced, stored in a retrieval system, transmitted or utilized in any form or by any means, electronic, mechanical, photocopying, recording or otherwise, without the prior permission of the copyright owner. Application for such permission should be addressed to the publisher.

Printed in India at Nice Printing Press, A-33/3A, Site-IV,
Industrial Area, Sahibabad, Ghaziabad, U.P.

Preface

Ageing is the process of growing old and is marked by the signs of changes in external appearance as well as internal functioning of the human body. To look young and feel fit with the passage of time, there is need to achieve self-grooming.

If you want to stay young, attractive and healthy, control ageing by keeping your body fit with the help of various techniques like slim and trim body, balanced diet, yoga, massage, exercise and latest medical facts with unpleasant side-effects.

Massage and exercise are vital ingredients of life and help you to lay firm ground to build a beautiful, slim and trim body. The book suggests many ways to remain young and healthy.

Pregnancy and menopause are important phases in a woman's life where a lot of care has to be taken to keep body healthy and youthful. Post-natal exercise programs, massage techniques, food habits and the art of make-up have been explained in this book to help you get back in shape and retain youthful look after pregnancy and childbirth.

Parvesh Handa

Contents

Contents

1

Know Your Body and Skin

Many of the questions we ask ourselves are about our own body. I have come across several men and women, some of them even going to be married or to conceive or near to the delivery of child. Many of such expectant mothers know least about the organs of their own body. Most of the teenagers feel hesitant to question about male or female genitals to their elders though their knowledge is very essential for everyone. It also allays fears and misconceptions.

ADOLESCENT PERIOD OF DEVELOPMENT

The teenage period between the age of twelve and twenty is considered to be the adolescent period of the life. Sex functions mature between 12 and 15 years of age in girls and 13 and 16 years in boys. In fact, this is the most important period of life, because it is the time when there is rapid growth and many sudden changes take place in physical, psychological and physiological development of the body. Girls tend to mature one to two years earlier than boys. Heredity factors play an important role in the development of body. Usually, at the onset of menstruation, a girl will be at the same age her mother was when she began to menstruate. It is seen that the girls tend to mature and menstruate early in summer climate. When menstruation starts, it is irregular for the first few months. The amount of flow varies widely. The periods become regular after two to three years. It may occur every two to three weeks or may occur only once in every two to three months and there is no need for any treatment. If a young girl is irregular in her periods after two years of start, she must consult a doctor for thorough examination.

A rectal examination will give the necessary information as to the state of the uterus and ovaries. It is not necessary to do a vaginal examination on such girls. Breasts usually begin to develop about one year before the onset of menstruation. It is common in a fair number of children when one breast or one nipple develops before the other. The unequal development of breasts means that one breast always remains larger than the other. The other breast will eventually catch up in its development and both breasts will be approximately of the same size in due course. During the developing stage of breasts, there is sometimes pain and tenderness. At about ten to twelve years of age, girls must be explained about the menstruation so that they are prepared for its onset. Parents should impart sex education to their growing children. The parents should instruct their children about adolescence, puberty and sexual changes. If the mother is not able to do it, then someone who is educated in the field, such as school teacher or a medical advisor should inform the child. It is best that a female child gets the information from mother or elder sister or from an older person rather than from her friends, who may be misinformed.

Following are the major evidences of puberty in male boys:

- Increase in the size of the external genitals.
- The appearance of pubic and underarm hair.
- The appearance of hair on the face and upper lip.
- Voice change, with deepening in tone.
- The development of muscles and masculine figure.

The major evidences of puberty in young females are the following:

- Breast development.
- The appearance of pubic and underarm hair.
- The assumption of the female types of figure.
- The onset of menstruation.

DEVELOPMENTAL CHANGES IN FEMALES

The organs such as the pituitary gland, the ovaries and testicles are responsible for the developmental changes of a child, because they begin to secrete larger quantities of the sex hormones and thus bring the changes seen in adolescence. Sometimes, breast enlargement is seen in a boy during puberty. There may be a nodule formed beneath the nipple at some time or other in boys between the age of eleven and fifteen years. This enlargement of the breast usually disappears spontaneously and requires no treatment. Both boys and girls tend to develop pimples and blackheads during adolescent period. This condition is called acne. Special diet, special methods of keeping the facial skin clean and correct medications prove helpful. This skin disorder among adolescents and teenagers has been described separately in this book. The parents should handle the psychological problems of adolescents carefully by providing assurance and encouragement, warmth, love and proper guidance to their children, who often are seen restlessness, disobedient, disrespectful and awkward during adolescence due to lack of important psychological changes that take place during this period.

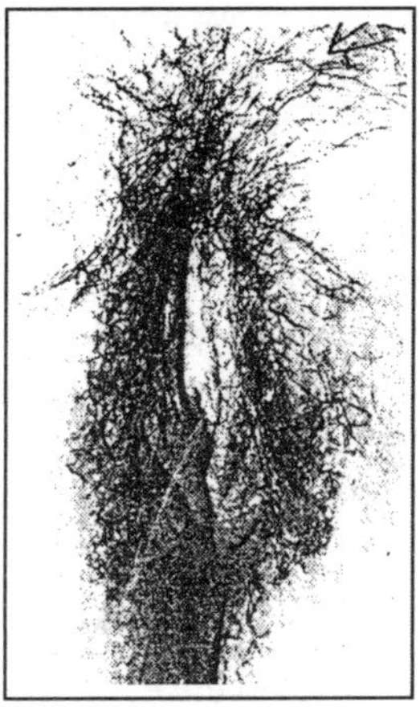

Female Genital Organ (outer view)

Most of the children have increased sexual urge during adolescence, which is a normal phenomenon and need not be discouraged. It is normal for boys and girls to want to get to know one another and get along each other. Sexual curiosity is a part of that desire to learn more about the opposite sex. During this period, sexual curiosity should be controlled gently and children should be directed so that their curiosity doesn't result in harmful pursuits. Now the question arises about the sex education among children. A child should be educated gradually from his or her earliest years when they start taking interest in sex. By the time adolescence is reached, children should know about sex so that they are better to manage their sexual urges. Ignorance about sexual matters often results in unwanted pregnancies or venereal infections among youngsters. It is natural for boys and girls to masturbate during adolescent period and the parents should not make them feel guilty about this practice. In most of the cases, in both boys and girls, late or delayed adolescence requires no treatment. In most of the cases, hormonal treatment is administered, which may leave a harmful effect due to a tendency towards slowing up of glandular function when the hormone treatment discontinues.

PHYSICAL GROWTH OF BOTH SEXES

Adolescence is the stage of life between childhood and adulthood usually beginning somewhere between the age 11 and 15 years. During adolescence, you experience many physical, mental, emotional and social changes. These changes prepare you to be an adult. Physical changes are a sign that a male or a female is going through the development stage called puberty.

Puberty is the time when you develop physical characteristics of adults of your own gender. During puberty, males' and females' bodies begin to change. These changes are a normal part of becoming a healthy adult. The chart below describes how male and female bodies change during puberty.

Males	Females
Male hormones production increases.	Female hormonal production increases.
Sudden, rapid growth occurs.	Sudden, rapid growth occurs.
All permanent teeth come into place	All permanent teeth grow.
Acne may appear.	Acne may appear.
Underarm hair appears.	Underarm hair appears.
Pubic hair appears.	Pubic hair appears.

Perspiration increases.	Perspiration increases.
External genital grow.	External genital grow.
Shoulders broaden.	Breasts develop.
Muscles develop.	Hips become wider.
Sperm production starts.	Body fat increases.
Facial hair appears.	Ovulation occurs.
Larynx gets larger and voice deepens	Menstruation starts.

ROLE OF HORMONES AND GLANDS IN HUMAN BODY

Hormones are one of the things that make your body change. Hormones are chemical substances produced in certain glands that help to regulate the way your body functions, and are produced by the organs of the endocrine system. The endocrine system is the system of glands throughout the body that regulate body functions. Each gland of the endocrine system makes one or more specific hormones. The pancreas makes the hormones to give insulin and glucagons. When the pancreas releases insulin into the blood, it lowers the level of sugar in the blood. When pancreas releases glucagons, it raises the blood sugar level. If the blood sugar is very low, you feel weakness and lightheaded. If it is too high, you can feel nauseated.

Role of the Endocrine System and Related Diseases

This system controls many of the changes in the body as below:

- **Parathyroid glands:** Located within the thyroid glands. They regulate the levels of calcium and phosphorus into the blood.
- **Adrenal glands:** Located on the top of kidneys that produce hormones and help regulate the balance of salt and water in the body. They also aid digestion and control body's response to emergencies and excitements.
- **Ovaries in female:** Female reproductive glands. Hormones produced in the ovaries control sexual development and the maturing of eggs.

- **Testes in male:** Male reproductive glands. Hormones produced in testes control sexual development and the production of sperm.
- **Pituitary gland:** Located at the base of the brain and produces several hormones that control the glands and organs such as thyroid glands, adrenal glands and kidneys. Pituitary gland hormones regulate the body's growth and development.
- **Thyroid gland:** Located alongside the trachea or windpipe. They regulate body growth and the rate of metabolism.
- **Pancreas:** Located behind the stomach and controls the level of sugar in the blood, and provide the small intestine with digestive chemicals called enzymes.

Menopause in Women?

Menopause or 'change of life' is a condition that usually occurs between the age group of 45 to 55. The menopause, sometimes, occurs in females in their twenties. The female reproductive time of life begins at adolescence in the early teens and continues until the beginning of the menopause. The symptoms of menopause are the following:

- Increased nervous tension.
- Menstrual disturbances.
- Hot flashes or chilly feelings.
- Excitability, easy fatigue and depression.
- Crying spells and sleeplessness.
- Palpitations, dizziness and frequent headaches.
- Numbness, tingling and other annoying symptoms.

These are the years when the lines and wrinkles settle more firmly unless the skin is regularly massaged and nourished with rich lubricating creams and moisturizing agents. Massage helps to keep the skin in good condition.

Male and Female Body Organs

- **The womb:** A compartment of female body in which the baby forms and grows till birth. It is also termed as uterus. A pear-shaped muscular organ situated deep in the lower abdomen usually of size 3''×2''×1'' when in non-pregnant state. It stretches gradually in size to store a fully formed baby. The lower part of the uterus is narrow and is called cervix with an opening in its tip.

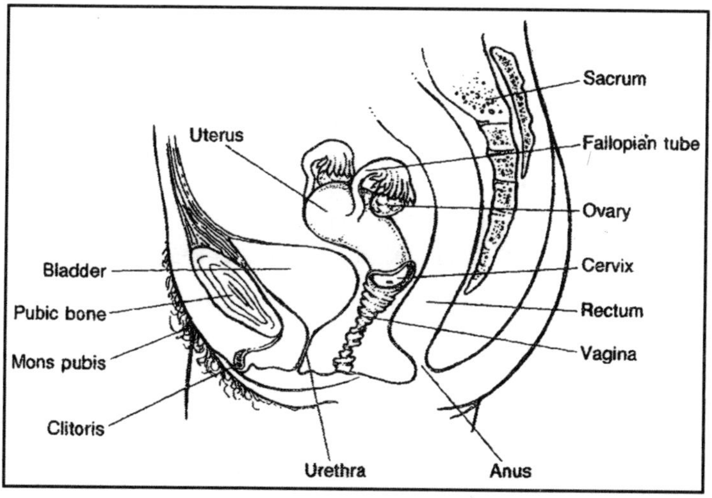

- **The cervix:** It protrudes into a long stretchable passage, which opens outside. The fluid containing sperms flows through this during sexual intercourse. The passage is called vagina.

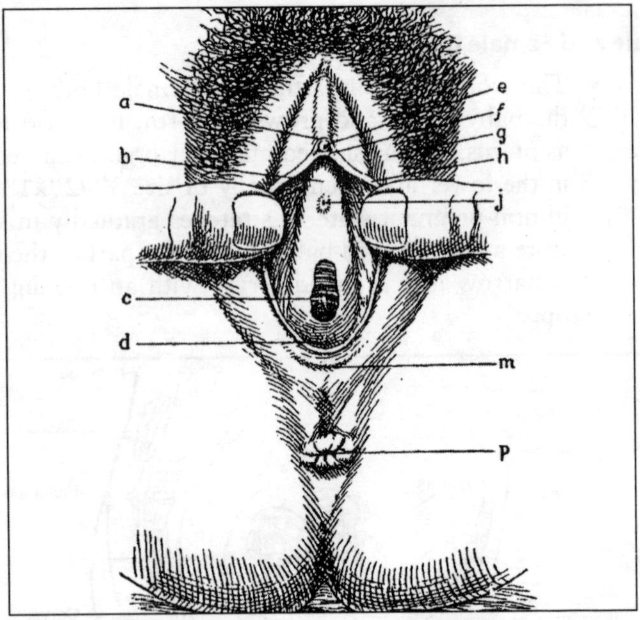

Female external genital organs

- **a.** Prepuce of the clitoris.
- **b.** Vestibule—anterior part.
- **c.** Orifice of the vagina.
- **d.** Vestibular fossa.
- **e.** Glans clitoridis.
- **f.** Frenulum.
- **g.** Labium mjus.
- **h.** Labium minus.
- **j.** Orifice of the urethra.
- **m.** Posterior commissure.
- **p.** Anus.

- **The vagina:** About 4" in length, vagina runs interiorly and caudally from the cervix between the bladder and rectum. It is directed from perennial opening upwards and backwards. Its upward end is closed.

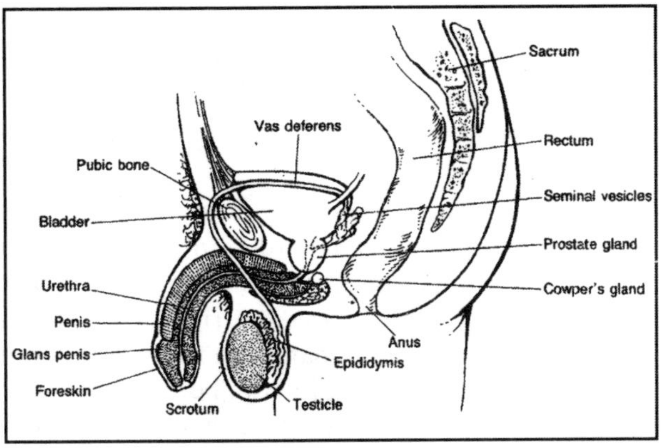

- **Uterus:** The pear-shaped uterus ranges from 2 to 3.3 cm in length and 0.5 to 1 cm in diameter. During pregnancy, the maximum dimensions of uterus are 8 cm in length, 5 cm in width and 4 cm in diameter. The upper broad end of uterus opens on either side into two long tubes called the fallopian tubes, each ending in a funnel-shaped opening guarded by five finger-like projections. The funnel-shaped opening lies close to the ovary on either side, which is a spherical, walnut- sized organ responsible for producing female hormones and eggs called ova. Ovulation occurs somewhere in the middle of a menstrual cycle, e.g. middle of an interval between two consecutive periods (roughly 14 days before any period). During a woman's reproductive life, only 400 ova are shed. When ovulation occurs, the ovum is picked up and travels down the fallopian tube towards the uterine cavity.
- **The penis:** The male genital organ, serves a dual function of erection and as a route of excretion of urine and semen. It is composed of three cylindrical structures of cavernous. The blood supply to the penis is primarily via the right and left internal arteries, which enter the base of the penis. Psychological factors account for most cases or cause of impotence. However, latest studies reveal that majority of cases of

impotence have organic reasons. Vasculogenic impotence is one of the most frequent causes for erectile failure generally due to poor arterial inflow into the penis or excessive venous leakage of the blood from the penis or both.

- **The liver:** The largest organ in the human body weighing approximately 1500 gm in an adult and lies in the right upper quadrant of the abdomen. The liver is divided in three lobes—the right, the left and the centre lobe. It has many important functions to perform and it is said to be a great chemical laboratory of the body. The liver is affected by a number of serious disorders, e.g. virus infections, parasites, disturbance of the circulation, stone formation in the bile duct due to poisonous substances and various kinds of food we eat after having been digested and absorbed from the gastro-intestinal tract. Various abnormalities of liver are liver cyst, jaundice, hepatitis, infections, serum, fatty liver, cirrhosis of the liver and liver cancer.
- **Gall bladder:** A small pear-shaped, muscular organ closely attached to the under surface of the liver varying in size and shape from person to person. The disorders of gall bladder include acute or chronic cholecystitis and jaundice. Sometimes, cancer occurs in the gall bladder.
- **Pancreas:** Pancreas is an important gland situated below the liver, which produces strong digestive juices necessary for assimilation of food. Pancreatitis is mild or very severe inflammation of the organ. Avoid taking alcohol in such condition; this may only aggravate the condition. Avoid stress as far as possible.
- **Urinary tract:** The human body is a living engine, which burns fuel (the food) and requires a constant supply of oxygen, water and various chemical substances to provide energy to the organs of body, repairing damaged tissues and keeping check on

kidneys. Normally, the body filters about 300 liters of fluid each day leaving approximately one litre of urine to be excreted from the body. The urine flows down the tiny tubules towards the centre of kidneys and finally, it is collected in the renal pelvis, from where it is eliminated from the body through the ureter and bladder. The common diseases of kidney are kidney infection, kidney stones, poly-cystic disease, bright's disease (nephritis), cancer of the urinary track, hydro-nephrosis, prostate gland, tuberculosis of the kidney, urethritis (inflammation) and uremia (toxic condition associated with kidney failure).

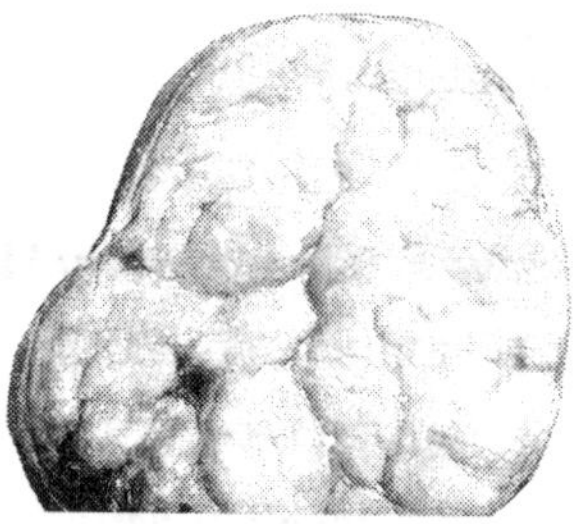

- **Ovary:** Ovaries have 1.5 inch length, 0.75 inch breadth and thickness resembles the egg of a pigeon in appearance, and is almond-shaped connected with the base of the uterus by means of the ligament tightly attached to fallopian tubes. The most common ovary disorders are amenorrhoea, hirsutism (unwanted hair on body), obesity and infertility. Poly-cystic ovarian diseases include functional cysts, follicular cyst, the corpus luted cyst, theca-luteal cyst, ovarian remnant syndrome (causing pelvic inflammatory disease or tumor), parovarian cysts, post-menopausal adnexal cysts, endometriosis (presence of tissue outside the uterus), torsion of the ovary associated with cysts or tumors, ovary cancer, epithelial tumors and neo-plastic lesions. All these diseases need immediate medical treatment.

The parts of male ejaculation system include:

- **Penis:** Made of a spongy tissue with many blood vessels.
- **Urethra:** Small tube that runs through the penis from the bladder. Urine and semen, at different times, leave the body through the urethra.

- **Scrotum:** A pouch that contains the testes.
- **Testes:** The glands that produce sperm and testosterone—the hormone that regulates male sexual development.
- **Prostate gland:** Produces fluids that protect sperm and move through the reproduction system.
- **Epididymis:** The collection of tubes is located next to testes to store sperms.

Adulthood

Around the age of 19, the stage called young adult begins. At this time, physical growth slows significantly, but young adults continue to grow mentally, emotionally and socially.

SKIN CARE

How to Balance a Dry Skin?

If your skin is dry?

If it feels tight, looks dull and perhaps is flaking?

If it lacks moisture and oil?

If more and more wrinkles appear on your face or body?

You should know the basics of self-care. The following care must be taken:

- Don't wash with hot water.
- Don't clean with soap.
- Use a moisturizer for a couple of times a day.
- Do not use artificial fragrances—they can hurt dry, sensitive skin.
- Of course, massage is the best remedy.

Guide to professional care:

- **Misting:** Spray your face with a fine mist of water—it is the best treatment for dry skin. For maximum benefits, you should always apply a moisturizer that contains humectants before misting through a bottle with a pump sprayer that emits a very fine spray that won't disturb make-up. You can also mix 10 drops of essential oil or a blend of oils in water. Some excellent oils to use are lavender, rose, chamomile, ylang-ylang and rose geranium. You should mist at least three times a day—morning, noon and evening.

- **Aromatherapy:** Daily use of warm facial compress using aromatherapy essential oils will greatly benefit dry skin by hydrating the skin and stimulating the water and oil glands. Essential oils such as lavender, rose and neroli are very gentle, harmonizing and balancing for the skin.
- **Nutritional supplements:** Skin supporting nutritional supplements can also help to heal dry skin. Here are few recommendations by the experts:
    1. Black currant oil (1,000-2,000 mg daily) is a rich source of omega-6 fatty acids, which are crucial for normal skin.
    2. Beta-carotine (15 mg a day taken twice in two parts each with lunch and dinner) is crucial for soft, smooth and disease-free skin.
    3. Zinc (15 mg daily with a meal) is important for repair of damaged skin tissue and its deficiency can cause dry skin.
    4. B-complex vitamin (100 mg a day after a meal) fulfils the deficiencies of thiamin, riboflavin, pantotheinic acid or biotin can lead to dry skin.
    5. Vitamin C (1,000 mg two to three times a day after meals) helps to immune system, which leads to healthier skin.
    6. Vitamin E (400 international units once or twice a day after meals) helps to replace cells on the skin's outer layer.

Normalizing an Oily Skin

If you have oily skin with medium to large pores, a shiny appearance and a tendency to have blackheads and blemishes—you may actually need more oil in your diet, the kind that contains fatty acids. There are two ways to deal with oily skin—externally and internally. Here are some treatments that alternative healers recommend:

- **Flaxseed oil:** Includes 1 to 3 teaspoons a day of flaxseed oil—oil rich in fatty acids. These fatty acids are found in vegetable oils and seed oils which are a must for healthy skin cells, no matter what type of skin you have.
- **Food:** Cut down on saturated fats. People who eat lot of red meat and dairy products, which are loaded with saturated fat can end up with oilier skin, clogged pores and more blemishes. So, for healthier skin, maximize fresh fruits, vegetables, whole grains, beans, nuts, seeds and fish. Minimize foods with saturated fat.
- **Aromatherapy:** Adding a drop of the essential oil of neroli to lavender, floral water and spraying the mixture on your skin several times a day is an excellent treatment for oily and overactive skin. Lavender tones and cleanses the skin. Neroli is considered a skin tonic. It penetrates the skin and helps to regulate the production of the sebum or oil.

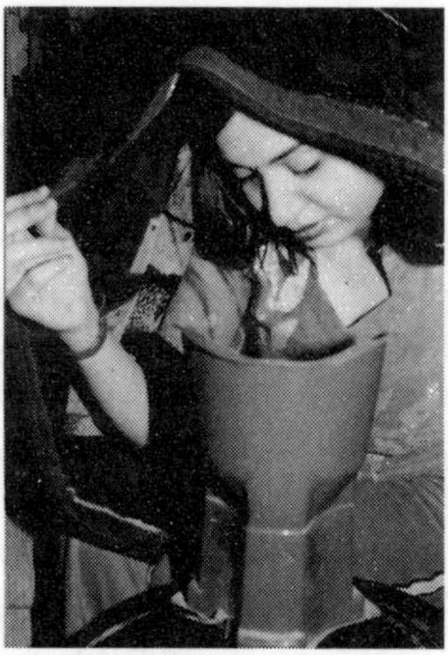

- **Herbs:** Herbal tea such as yarrow, sage and peppermint removes leftover cleanser and dirt from the oily skin.
- **Steaming the face:** Steaming helps to deep-clean oily skin. Steam the face for 5 to 8 minutes once or twice a week. After steaming, rinse with warm water, then splash with cool water and pat dry. Warm water activates the oil glands, while cooler water slows them down.

A Wrinkled Skin

Age group	Type and care required
Below 16	Usually the skin is clear, smooth and youthful.
17-20	Usually the skin is clear. Use moisturizing lotion.
21-25	Usually the skin is clear and smooth. Use only moisturizer and cleansing milk before sleep at night to remove dirt.
26-30	These are the peak years for a woman to take care of the skin. Use only moisturizing lotion, foundation cream and light make-up.
31-40	During these years, the first fine lines begin to appear. The skin texture usually becomes drier if not cared properly. Use heavy moisturizer under the make-up.
41-55	These are the years when the fine lines settle more firmly. Give regular massage and nourish with rich lubricating creams. Facial helps to keep the skin in good condition.
56 and above	Avoid excess use of soap. Treat skin gently. Avoid too hot or too cold water on the skin. No hard massaging. Skin-firming preparations will help a lot.

PHYSIOLOGICAL EFFECTS OF MASSAGE

To obtain best results from a facial or scalp massage, one must have a thorough knowledge of all the structures involved, e.g. the muscles, the nerves and the blood vessels. Every muscle or a nerve has a motor point. The position of motor points will vary in individuals due to difference in body structure. The

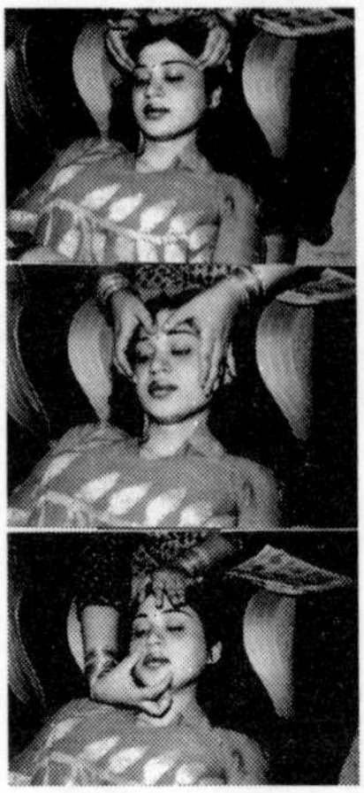

massage activates, circulation, secretion, nutrition and excretion of the skin. There are several beneficial results such as nourishment of skin at all structures, reduction of fat cells in subcutaneous tissues, flexibility and softness of skin, increase in circulation of blood, stimulation of activity of skin glands, strengthening of the skin's fiber muscles, soothing and refreshing of nerves of skin and pain. The frequency of the facial or scalp massage depends upon the age and condition of the skin to be treated. If the skin is in excellent condition, a weekly massage is sufficient.

Remember, when indulging in a facial massage try to relax, speak softly or as far as possible keep silent and massage in a quiet environment, maintain utmost cleanliness, make sure your hands are not very cold or warm before touching the skin and the nails of your fingers should not be too long or pointed. All self-massage movements must be made in the direction of the lymphatic circulation, e.g. towards the heart. When you massage arms or legs, movements must go upwards from extremities towards the trunk. Do not massage yourself if you are suffering from fever, heart ailments, disorder of the blood vessels, a skin disease, varicose veins, vascular lesions and passing through seventh month of pregnancy.

CORRECTING A FLUSHED COMPLEXION

Deep in the skin are nerves, blood vessels, sweat glands giving off waste matter and sebaceous glands, which supply oil for lubricating the skin (and the hair). Sebaceous glands almost always lead directly into hair follicles, which is why hair has a natural grease of its own. The material for making all these and for the new cells which make up the skin are supplied from the food we eat. Diet which is essential for a lovely skin includes eggs, milk, butter, cream and cheese, lean meat, fish, fresh fruit and leafy green vegetables.

Blood cells carry nourishment and oxygen to every part of the body and of course, to the skin. If your diet is lacking in vitamins and minerals, the nourishment will be poor. If you are breathing in stale, stuffy air, the quality of oxygen reaching your skin will be poor. Each time you fill your lungs with pure fresh air, you are giving yourself a free beauty treatment. That wonderful glow you have when you come in from a brisk walk and your skin is tingling more than just a marvelous feeling of vitality, bringing nourishing supplies to every inch of your body and carrying away waste.

Your skin is sensitive and as finely tuned as a barometer, which records facts about you in much the same way. Poor diet, lack of sleep, nervous upsets—all these react on your complexion as spots, shadows under your eyes and lines. If you become very tired, you cannot prevent your face showing it and your skin will droop into folds of weariness and your eyes become dull and heavy. Some faces have a tendency to be red and flushed complexion. Consult a doctor. If there is no underlying medical problem to explain the red, flushing appearance, it is probably that you simply have a ruddy complexion. It cannot be permanently altered. Over exposure to sun, steam baths, hot foods and alcohol should be avoided since they may exaggerate the redness. If regular cosmetics may prove ineffective, you may want to try one of the under make-up toners, which can be applied as a film under regular make-up for they help to even out skin colour tones.

How to Improve your Complexion?

The physical assets are most important for every woman, especially for working women. However, just a fair complexion is not as important as the overall personality, height, figure and communication ability. If you have a pleasing manner and smart figure, there is no reason why you will not be successful in your career. Be sure that the colour of your skin will be no reason in your getting a position.

Discolouration of skin is common among women. It is often mistaken for scarring. Initially, all scars are red, pink or purple. This colour fades over the next year. The blood vessels in a scarred area may be very noticeable. All colour changes can be camouflaged with make-up or special covering cream and many scars become temporarily lumpy during healing and later flatten. The skin may darken because of pigment deposited in the skin, which are iron and melanin. Colour cells (melanocytes) are studded in millions throughout the skin and they produce a brown pigment called melanin. All races have the same number of colour cells in the skin but they produce different amounts of pigments and the colour production increases by sunshine.

The colour of the skin also depends on the blood supply to the skin. An extensive network of blood vessels runs underneath the epidermis and they react to heat and cold. The skin, too, reacts to heat and cold in many ways. Most of the reactions are to the body's advantages, but some are troublesome and a few are dangerous. The body needs a constant internal temperature for all its processes to function properly. The skin regulates the body temperature by reducing loss of heat when the outside is cold or losing extra heat when the body is too hot. We, too, assist the skin in doing this by altering our clothing. In hot weather, warm clothes or a fever can cause the body temperature to rise and set off the heat losing mechanism of the skin such as reddening of the skin due to enlarging of the blood vessels, swelling of the skin and sweating. The body cools itself by evaporating the sweat from the skin. This is the most important way of losing heat.

Many skin diseases especially eczema provoke the colour cells of the skin to overproduce pigments, which drop down into the dermis of the skin and leave brown marks when the skin trouble disappears. This is called post-inflammatory hyper-pigmentation. Fortunately, the body can slowly remove this pigment and most darkening fades over 1 to 2 years. The darkening is worst in black skin and may occur even after acne. Once this type of colour change has developed, only with passage of time it can be removed. The early treatment of the disease will also help to prevent the colour change.

Increased hormone levels in the body during pregnancy stimulate the colour cells of the face and the brown patches appearing specially around the eyes, on cheeks and on the upper lip. The contraceptive pill can cause similar brown patches. Hormones occurring naturally cause this problem mostly in women especially those of mediterranean origin who are not on the pill or are pregnant, but rarely in men. The brown patches last for several months and then slowly fade away. It is most important to avoid sunshine, which will darken the existing patches. You should also use sun-screen lotion after consulting a skin specialist over the brown patches together with a sunshade or sunhat.

Allergies to perfume may produce dark patches on the face and the neck. These perfumes are present in after-shaves, cosmetics and creams, in addition to perfume sprays. It is important to wash off all perfumes before sunbathing. Very dark patches may develop in later life in the groins and armpits. They can also be signs of illness so get them checked by a doctor.

CARING THE SKIN

Skin Prone to Sunburn

Excessive exposure to sun permanently damages the skin and leads to harmful effects such as premature ageing, wrinkling, discolouration, leathery texture and cancerous skin conditions. To protect damages and discolouration of the skin complexion several products are available in the market.

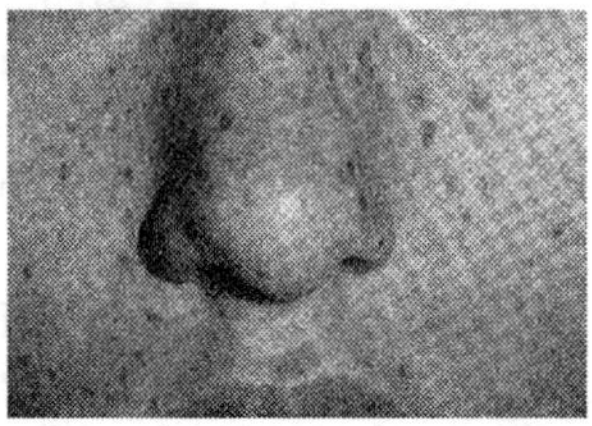

Sun's burning rays are most intense between 11 a.m. and 3 p.m. No sunburn is likely to take place before 8 in the morning and after 4 p.m. The skin damaged by burning or severe inflammation always leaves scars. Surface injuries often heal with temporary discolouration only if burning is not very severe. The face heals quickly and scars are often unnoticeable. Plastic surgery, if done carefully along the expression lines, makes the scars invisible. The backs of the hands heal well, the arms less well and the legs slowly with bad scarring. The chest and the upper back may produce unpleasant scars due to the burns, which take weeks to heal and the scars gape and widen. Minor blemishes or birth-marks should never be removed from these areas for cosmetic reasons, as the scars will become worse than the blemish.

Though the sunrays are very important for keeping the skin healthy, sunburn is extremely harmful to the skin. Infrared rays of the sun are hot and bring warmth to the body, which is essential for our health. But the skin gets burnt due to excessive ultra-violet rays.

Melanin under the skin prevents the skin from getting burnt and that is the reason the blondes and dark-complexioned people get less sunburns than the fair-complexioned people. This is because the darker the skin, the quantity of melanin in the body is more. The ill effects of sunrays is maximum on children between the age 6 to 8 years, in women between 25 to 30 years of age and men between 30 to 35 years. Ultra-violet rays destroy the melanin in the body and the skin gets darkened, the rays cut the skin and cracks it and the result is drying of the skin. As a result, the skin swells and rashes appear on it. Then fresh melanin comes out and the skin gets blackened.

Sunburn reaction on the body is the same as the burning of the skin by steam and very hot oil. It results in the skin getting dried, the blood vessels get swollen, and the cells are damaged. Ordinary sunburn can be cured within three to four days but a strong sunburn creates rashes and the skin peels off in layers, new cells are born and a new skin does appear again, but it is much more dry and thick as compared to original one. The new skin is often brown in colour and cracks, and wrinkles easily. Such wrinkles are hard to cure. You may benefit from a cold bath if you are suffering from sunburn. Avoid using soap. Protect the skin from hot sun-rays until the sunburn is cured. If rashes appear, consult a skin specialist. The degree of tolerance of sun depends upon the nature of the skin. Direct hot sunrays are more harmful in the month of June when the sun gets nearest to the earth. When you go out in the sun, drink as much water as you can for a cooling effect.

Caring the Skin in Different Seasons

Following steps are essential to treat skin in different seasons:

Summer Care:

- Wash the face with soap (preferably washing gel) at least twice a day.
- Cleanse the face before sleep at night to remove dust or stale make-up.
- Apply astringent lotion if the skin is excessively oily.
- Wash the face and bathe with cold water.
- Perform a home facial once a week.

Winter Care:

- Avoid using soap as far as possible.
- Clean the face before going to bed at night.
- Wash the face once a day with tepid water.
- Perform a home facial once a fortnight.
- Apply a rich cream and moisturizer at night or when going out in cold.
- If your skin is excessively dry, apply a vitamin face cream.

Monsoon Care:

- A three steps skin care program: Cleansing, toning and moisturizing should be made part of your daily routine.
- Even an oily skin needs moisturizer. Lack of moisturizer enhances the tell tale lines giving an impression of older age.
- Moisturize the area around your eyes daily at night. Wipe off excess cream after 30 minutes. This will ensure your eyes are not puffy the next morning.
- Steam the face at least once a week if your skin is blemished. Steam the face before massage to unclog the pores.

REGULAR HOME FACIAL

The first step in caring for your skin externally is cleansing. Perspiration, grease, dust, stale make-up, dirt and bacteria all collect on your skin and must be removed completely. You must clean the skin with cleansing milk, cream, lotion or just plain cold cream and then remove cleanser with tissues, damp cotton wool or a small Turkish towel. You should always follow your cleansing routine by toning your skin with a mild skin freshener, a strong astringent lotion or with a medium strength skin tonic. You must remember that toning removes greasiness remaining from cleansing preparations, closes pores and refines the skin if you intend to do make-up and it leaves a clean smooth texture, which hold foundation and powder for a much longer time. Nourishing is an essential part of any beauty routine except for very young skin. Dirt, dust, hot and cold weather, cosmetics and even sunlight—all tend to dry out the skin robbing it off moisture and oil. The skin foods attempt to put back some of the nourishment. It is not necessary to use a thick heavy skin food every night. If you do not like a greasy face before going to bed, then it is easy to choose a light easily absorbed skin food, which will disappear in minutes. Many of the new liquid skin foods come into this category. If you feel you need a richer heavier cream, then use it when you are having the bath.

Facial is the quickest way of reviving faded skin, livening and refining complexion. It leaves the skin soft, smooth and glowing with vitality. The most luxurious way of having a facial is to go to a beauty saloon. This will help to do a thorough job of relaxing jangled nerves so that you emerge feeling fresher, looking younger and beautifully relaxed. If you get no time or you cannot afford the luxury of regular saloon treatment, then the best thing is to give yourself a facial at home. Choose a time when you can be undisturbed and quiet. Always get everything ready before you start so that you can relax and enjoy it. A regular facial once a fortnight is a good habit, which will ensure you a youthful and fresh skin for a long time. For a quick home facial, following routine should be done:

- Tie your hair away from the face and the neck or wear a hair-band.
- Cleanse your face and neck with cleansing milk and wipe off first with a facial tissue, then with a wet towel.
- Apply cream in dots all over the face and blend it thoroughly. Then massage your face and neck in upward direction.
- Prepare a face pack suited to your skin type and apply on your face. When it is dry, wash your face and neck with cool water keeping your eyes closed. Dry your skin and apply skin tonic.
- If you have an important date, use skin tonic after facial. Then apply moisturizer and make-up.

You should choose a face pack suited for your skin. Mask is an effective beauty treatment. On a thorough clean face spread fairly thick layer of mask of your choice avoiding the area of the mouth and circle around the eyes. Then lie on your back and keep the mask on for 15 to 20 minutes till the time it is dry. Remove the mask with warm water and absorbent cotton or tissues. Keep slices of peeled cucumber on your eyes when having a mask on the face. You must not talk after you have applied the face mask.

Facial for Acne Skin

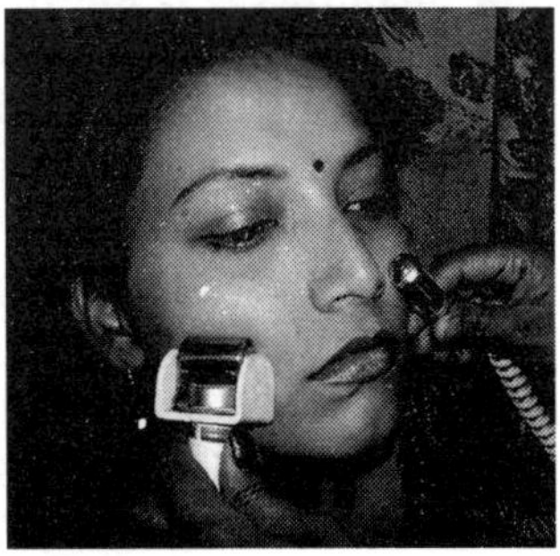

Acne is common in teens and twenties and it is a serious disorder of the sebaceous glands, which requires medical direction. To keep the skin conditions under control, observe the following conditions:

- Reduce the oiliness of the skin.
- Remove blackheads.
- Regular cleansing of the skin.
- Use of special medicated preparations.
- Have a well-balanced regular diet.

Home facial for acne skin should be done like this:

- Cleanse the face with medicated soap and warm water. Seek advice of a skin specialist for use of a suitable soap.
- Apply acne cream or ointment all over the face and the neck.
- Apply high frequency current over the affected skin for not more than five minutes. Then remove acne cream with tissue paper.
- Apply suitable face pack and keep it on for ten minutes.
- Remove the mask and blot the residue with a cold or wet towel.
- Saturate cotton swab with astringent lotion and apply with a lime blotting movement.
- Moisten a piece of cotton with an antiseptic lotion and touch each and every pimple or acne.
- Never apply make-up on acne skin.

Usually, all teenagers have some acne varying from a few blackheads to a very unsightly and upsetting problem of large pus-filled spots. Steaming is beneficial to clean all types of skin. It cleans the skin, stimulates the circulation and unclogs blocked pores. Electrical devices are available to produce steam and this process is known as sauna facial. If your skin is dry, steam your face once in a week. In case of an oily skin, the steaming can be done daily but not more than five minutes. Steam the face by leaning over a large bowl of boiling water after having covered your head with a towel, making the tent around the bowl. Do not get too close to the boiling water for if the steam is too hot, it might cause broken veins. There are many preparations for acne like lotions, gels, creams, ointments, scrubs and soaps available in market today. Peeling of skin unblocks the pores, which helps blackheads and small spots. Antibiotic lotions are successful in treating acne, but it takes about two months to work your doctor's advice is must.

SKIN CLEANSING, TONING, MOISTURIZING AND NOURISHING

These are the first and among the most important of the skin care products. Soap is a cleanser although not very good one when it comes to cleansing skin especially when the make-up has been used. If you must have to use soap, choose a mild one—baby soap or a type specially designed for the face. But in addition to your soap and water, you will still need to use a cosmetic cleanser as well if you are to cleanse your skin thoroughly and care for it properly.

Cosmetic cleansers are made in many forms and these include ordinary cold cream, cleansing creams, liquefying creams, cleansing milks and lotions, liquid cleansers often designed especially for dry or oily skins. All cleansers will dissolve make-up and remove dirt, dust and grime from the pores. Some are slightly astringent or refreshing and these are usually intended for quick daytime cleansing before reapplying fresh make-up. The creams and emulsions are more commonly used at night when it is essential to deep cleanse the skin to remove every trace of make-up and grime. On the whole, almost any cleanser will do for any type of skin but generally the rich creams are best for dry skins and the liquefying creams or cleansing lotions are best for the oily type of skin. There are special cleansers made for blemished skins and these tend to have a drying effect.

Use of Toning Preparations

These are intended to close pores, freshen the complexion and refine the skin. There are many different types and one kind or another should be used after cleansing and before making up to ensure a smooth matt make-up and also after cleansing and before applying skin food at night. Toning products include skin fresheners, skin tonics, astringent lotions and milk, various flower extracts, herbal and camphor lotions and also witch hazel and rose water. If you have a dry skin, you should use a mild toning lotion such as skin freshener or a flower water such as rose water or one of the flower lotions.

Normal skins can generally use any brand of skin tonic or skin freshener while oily skin often benefit from an astringent lotion or one of the herbal or camphor lotions or astringent milk. Although an astringent will close up and prevent oiliness seeping through make-up, yet care should be taken not to choose a lotion, which is too astringent otherwise this may stimulate the sebaceous glands into producing yet more oil.

Moisturizing the Skin

These are often included among the nourishing creams but in fact they are intended to do a different job for the most part and so can fit into a category of their own. Most moisturizing creams and lotions have low oil but high moisture content. Although they supply some moisture to the skin, they work mainly by preventing evaporation of natural moisture from the skin. They protect the skin by combating the drying effects of cold weather, sun, hair dryers, central heating, radiant fire, dust, fog and tinted cosmetics.

Almost all skins need moisturizer, even oily types, but for the dry or mature skin, a moisturizer is vital. The drier your skin the more lavish you should be with your use of moisturizer either in cream or liquid form. Apply it after cleansing and toning and always before making up or use it on its own—and reapply frequently during the day—if you are not wearing make-up. A thin film of moisturizer is helpful under a face pack for a dry skin and it can be used in place of a skin food on a young skin or a youthful normal or oily skin, which needs some nourishment.

Using Nourishing Preparations

These include all skin foods whether they are oil-based or of moisturizing type and whether they are light and immediately absorbed or heavy and sticky, needing to be massaged into the skin. Hormone creams and lotions, vitamin products, serum ampoules, anti-wrinkle creams and lotions, biologically-active preparations containing placental extracts and other laboratory-prepared ingredients all come into the nourishing group.

What your skin needs will depend on its type and age. The more dry and the more mature it is, the richer or the more active product is required. It is hard to generalize but on average, the ordinary inexpensive skin foods will supply all that the skin needs in the way of oils and lubricating ingredients throughout the 20s and 30s and possibly until the menopause.

During the menopause and afterwards when the body's supply of hormones and other vital elements slow down then creams and lotions containing hormones and other special extracts and serums, rich creams containing vitamins and concentrated oils may all help to give the skin a more youthful appearance. Many of these are, however, expensive because they are the result of long research in expensively maintained laboratories but often a single course is sufficient to have effect for some months.

DISORDERS OF SKIN

To obtain proper results from a massage, one must not only have a thorough knowledge of all the structures involved—the muscles, the nerves and the blood vessels, pressure points on the skin, a skillful massage techniques, frequency of massage movements on a particular type of skin, conditions to be treated and above all, the health of the skin to be massaged is very important for excellent results. There are several disorders of the skin, which mar a beautiful skin. Some of the common skin disorders are described here, which harm a beautiful skin.

DISCOLOURATION OF SKIN

Discolouration of skin is often mistaken for scarring. Initially, all scars are red, pink or purple. This colour fades over the next year. The blood vessels in a scarred area may be very noticeable. All colour changes can be camouflaged with make-up or special covering cream and many scars become temporarily lumpy during healing and later flatten. The skin may darken because of pigments deposited in the skin, which are iron and melanin.

Colour cells (melanocytes) are studded in millions throughout the skin and they produce a brown pigment called melanin. All races have the same number of colour cells in the skin but they produce different amounts of pigment and the colour increased by sunshine. The colour of the skin also depends on the blood supply to the skin. An extensive network of blood vessels runs underneath the epidermis and they react to heat and cold. The skin too reacts to heat and cold in many ways. Most of the reactions are to the body's advantage, but some are troublesome and a few are dangerous. The body needs a constant internal temperature for all its processes to function properly. The skin regulates the body temperature by reducing loss of heat when the outside temperature is cold or losing extra heat when the body is too hot. We too assist the skin in doing this by altering the clothing. In hot weather, warm clothes cause the body temperature to rise and set off the heat losing mechanism of the skin such as reddening of the skin due to enlarging of the blood vessels, swelling of the skin and sweating. The body cools itself by evaporating the sweat from the skin.

Many skin diseases especially eczema provoke the colour cells of the skin to over produce pigments which drop down into the dermis of the skin and leave brown marks when the skin trouble disappears. This is called post-inflammatory hyper-pigmentation. Fortunately, the body can slowly remove this pigment and most darkening fades over in one to two years. The darkening is worst in dark skin and may occur even after acne. The early treatment will help to prevent the colour change.

Increased hormone levels in the body during pregnancy stimulate the colour cells of the face and the brown patches appearing specially around the eyes, on cheeks and on the upper lip. The contraceptive pills can cause similar brown patches. Hormones occurring naturally cause this problem mostly in women who are not on the pills or are pregnant but rarely in men. The brown patches last for many months and then slowly fade away. It is most important to avoid sunshine, which will darken the existing patches. You should also use sun-blocking cream with the consultation of a skin specialist over the brown patches together with a sunshade or sunhat.

Allergies to a perfume may also produce dark patches on the face and on the neck. These perfumes are present in after-shave lotions, cosmetics and creams, in addition to perfume sprays. It is important to wash off all perfumes before sunbathing. Very dark patches may develop in the groins and armpits in later life. They can also be signs of illness so get them checked by a doctor.

Three Ages of the Skin

- **Infancy**: In babies and infants, skin bacteria can break down urine to produce ammonia, which is very irritating to the skin and may cause a nappy rash. This forms sores and ulcers on the skin. It is very important to wash the skin at each nappy change to remove bacteria. Many babies are prone to getting a rash, which often looks like a bad nappy rash but also affects the creases of the bottom and is very red and crusted all over the bottom. This is a form of eczema, known as seborrhoeic eczema of infancy. It needs the usual protective creams for baby's bottoms—zinc and castor oil, drapolene, etc. Avoid use of baby detergents and soaps. There are detergent-free emulsifying ointments or aqueous creams available from the chemists for washing infants. Many times the rash become infected with thrush and small pustules are visible. Babies who are kept too warm and become damp from sweating and urine often develop red spots, which may blister usually in the folds. Milk spots may be a cause of alarm in lactating mothers especially with the first babies and the infants. They are tiny spots, which appear on cheeks, normally between the ages of 2 to 6 weeks and soon disappear. Infancy is also the age when atopic eczema starts.
- **Adolescence**: The major affliction of adolescence is the tendency to develop acne, which affects every teenager when the puberty starts. It is important to take acne seriously and to treat it quickly to prevent scarring. Another problem may be the enlargement of birthmarks or an increased awareness of birthmarks, at the time of developing relationship with opposite sex. Male pattern baldness may also develop in late

teenage years and is a further affront to young male vanity. Rapid growth of height may give rise to stretch marks on the trunk, abdomen and limbs—which may further get worsened by additional physical stress (weight-bearing).

- **Ageing**: As we age, the skin becomes thinner both in the outer layer and in the supporting tissue resulting in wrinkled skin, which becomes less elastic. This is increased by exposure to sun so is often noticeable initially on the neck and face (with yellowish lumps with a scraggy appearance). The blood vessels lose some support and bruising occurs. Over bathing, especially with foam bath may give a very dry and itchy skin. Older skin tends to develop lumps and bumps — warts, skin tags, freckles, white patches and skin cancers. Hair thinning may occur all over the scalp.

Acne Marks, Scars and Skin Blemishes Making Skin Aged

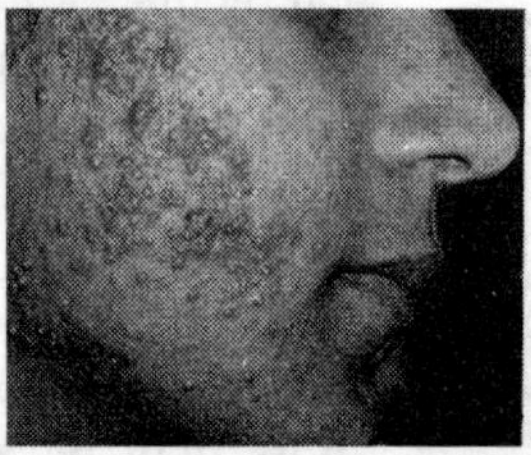

A scar is raised or indented section of fibrous tissue formed by the body's healing process in response to an injury that penetrates the skin. If the injury penetrates, only in the top layer of the skin (the epidermis), the healing process may leave only a light, temporary marks. But if the injury penetrates the body's deeper layer of skin (the dermis), then the body may form a scar. Besides cuts, scrapes and burns, picking a pimple or scratching a chicken pox sore can also leave a scar. The following measures are adopted to prevent scar:

- If the scar is lighter or redder than the rest of the skin of your body, application of a good foundation cream can eliminate it.
- Apply a topical antibiotic once a wound is clean and bleeding has stopped. Smear on an antibacterial ointment after consulting a doctor.

- Take Vitamin C, which can speedily healing of a wound that may cause a scar.

Blemishes are clogged pores consisting of dead skin cells, oil secreted by tiny sebaceous glands in the skin that produces bacteria. There are three types of blemishes lasting for three to four weeks: blackhead or whiteheads, papules and cysts. Blackheads and whiteheads develop close to the surface of the skin. With a blackhead, the oil and accumulated debris forces the pore open the oil oxidized to black. A whitehead is similar to blackhead, but is closed in which the oil and debris remain beneath the skin surface. A papule is a red bump that occurs because of an inflammation under the skin at a hair follicle. Cysts occur deeper within the pores in the form of swollen red or white papules. There are several remedies to get rid of blemishes:

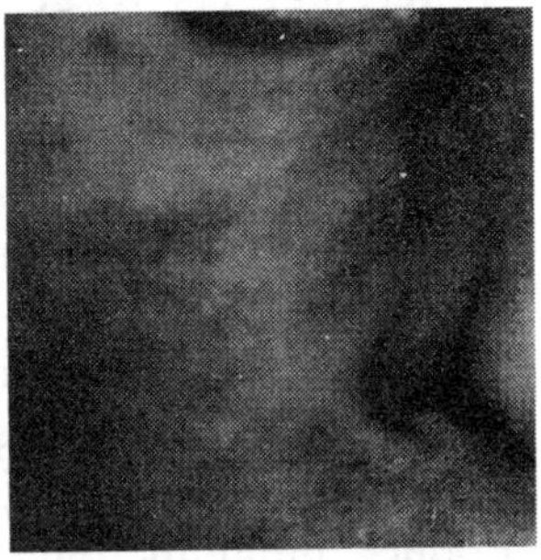

- A good treatment for emerging pimple is to apply ice. Wrap an ice cube in a washcloth and hold it to the pimple for five minutes. Cooling it will decrease inflammation.
- Products with benzoyl peroxide can help get rid of blemishes and prevent new ones from forming.
- Blemish cover cream is designed to use with regular cover creams. Let it set for a couple of minutes, then apply foundation cream for deep coverage.

Skin Cancer Making Skin Texture Look Aged

The skin tumour is caused by excessive exposure of sunrays and in case it is not treated in time it leads to skin cancer. Avoid excess exposure to X-rays. Keratosis is another form of skin cancer in old age when numerous scaly patches appear on the scalp and other areas such as face, ear and back of the hands. Fleshy, rapidly growing lumps or bumps in the skin may spread to the other parts of the body and should be dealt with immediately. Skin cancer rarely spreads to the rest of the body but needs to be removed by an experienced surgeon through radiotherapy or surgery or cryotherapy—a process in which liquid nitrogen can be used to kill cancer cells by freezing. Try to get skin cancer diagnosed earliest by an experienced doctor. It is easier to treat it at an early stage.

There are several types of skin lightening creams or bleaching creams available in the market. They all contain chemicals (usually hydroquinone), which interfere with the production of melanin. These creams cannot lighten the post-inflammatory pigmentation, which is the common cause of brown patches. They can lighten the normal skin, birth marks and freckles. It is generally very irritating to the skin and produce inflammation with more darkening of the skin or blotchy discolouration. In case of itching and redness, stop using bleaching creams immediately as sometimes the chemicals in it may damage the underlying tissues leaving black lumps and cysts or can cause permanent colour loss.

Stains, Marks and Patches

- **Port wine stains:** These are flat, red marks usually found on the face and scalp. They cannot be removed through surgery. These should be treated by laser treatment and infrared treatment. They can be camouflaged.
- **Strawberry marks:** They are developed soon after the baby is born and grow rapidly from a bluish small mark to bluish-red fleshy lump of blood vessels. They can bleed also. The mark increases in size very fast but eventually it shrinks. By the age of ten only a white scar remains. Avoid surgical treatment for it will cause a worse scar in the end.
- **Birth marks:** Some babies have red birth mark on the nape of the neck, which is usually covered by hair.
- **Dark patches:** Very large areas of brown hairy thickening may develop on the arms and the trunk in the teens. It is not possible to remove them as large scars are left and these reappear after a short time.

- **Mangolian spots:** These occur in babies. They may have bluish birth marks over the lower back. These are harmless and usually fade after 18 to 24 months.
- **Skin tags:** These are small tags of skin very common on the neck, in the armpits and groins. They can be removed by tying fine thread around the stalk. They can be snipped off with scissors or burnt.
- **Seborrhoeic warts:** By the age of 60, sometimes lots of greasy warts appear on the face, neck and trunk. Very often, people worry about them as being skin cancers. They may become itchy and sore. These may be removed by scraping or freezing.

2

The Magic of Hands to Fight Ageing

MASSAGE FOR AGEING SKIN

There are two types of skin ageing: intrinsic and extrinsic, and both contribute to wrinkling. Intrinsic ageing is something that happens as the genes inherited from the parents trigger a reduction of two connective fibers: collagen and elastin. Collagen supports the skin and elastin gives it flexibility. Together collagen and elastin give skin its structure and tone. After age of 30, connective fibers start to break down and the skin starts to become more lax. Extrinsic ageing is ageing that comes from environmental factors, especially sun damage.

If you want to know how much genetics contributes to skin ageing and how much damage is caused by the sun, just look at the top of your forearm, then flip it over and check out the underside. Genetics is responsible for the skin on the underside, whereas sun exposure is responsible for the skin on top. The invisible sunrays penetrate below the skin surface and encourage wrinkles, because they damage connective fibers. These are the same rays that stimulate production of melanin and produce a tan, a look that makes looking young and sexy.

You need to think about the future of your skin getting prematurely older. Try to prevent more damage from occurring. The power of massage prevents most of what we don't like about our skin. Before we discuss in detail about massage—the magic of hands, here are a few natural tips to avoid premature wrinkling:

How to Avoid Wrinkles?

- **Daily care**
  1. Wash the face with a foaming cleanser.
  2. Smoothing on an alpha hydroxy acid lotion that removes old cells and uncovers new ones.
  3. Stroking on a sunscreen that also doubles as a moisturizer.
  4. Care when applying make-up. Remember, excessive make-up is very harmful for the skin.
- **Alpha hydroxy acid (AHA) treatment**

  To erase fine wrinkles and prevent more from forming, make AHA the foundation of your daily skin care regimen. These acids are derived from sugarcane, fruit and milk. They loosen old wrinkles cells on the skin's surface, peel them off, then uncover the younger, fresher cells underneath. They also plump the skin's surface—in essence, filling in the dents that you notice as wrinkles. AHA available in the market in lotion, cream or gel form, usually has moisturizing properties. Gels are recommended to younger women who do not need the moisturizing properties of lotions. Lotions are recommended to those who need a lightweight moisturizer and creams are for those who need a heavier moisturizer to keep their skin from drying out and causing tiny lines just from the dryness. Test before applying an AHA preparation. To test, smear a drop of a 5% AHA preparation on a small section of skin under jaw. If there is no sign of redness or irritation by the next day, go ahead with the preparation. For this treatment, wash your face, pat it dry, apply an AHA preparation to your face, then apply your usual sunscreen. Smooth the AHA preparation over your entire face, but not closer to your eyes. If there is no irritation for several days, you can increase use of AHA to twice a day: once in the morning and once at night.

- **Use of sunscreen**

  People when they plan to spend the day are recommended to use two sunscreens at the same time to protect their face against wrinkle-forming forces and ultra-violet rays (UVR) which penetrate to the deeper layer of the skin.

- **Keep weight steady**

  Gaining and losing even small amount of weight can create fine wrinkles by the constant stretching and tightening of skin. Try to avoid frequent weight-gain.

Massage to Fight Ageing and Wrinkles

Massage is one of the easiest ways for attaining and maintaining health, youth, vigour and beauty. Aches, pains, insomnia (lack of sleep), tension and stress can be alleviated with a simple instrument—hands. Many experts advise couples to touch each other more often as this can prevent physical and mental illness in a human body. Massage has the following effects on the body:

- Improves circulation.
- Relaxes muscles.
- Aids digestion by stimulating the lymphatic system.
- Eliminates the waste products and toxins in the body.
- Provides energy.
- Refreshes and revitalizes the body.

Massage is the oldest form of medical treatment in 19th century. Early morning massage just after waking up has a miraculous effect on the various organs. Massage is incorporated in Naturopathic and Yogic treatments—an Indian system of medicine dating back to 1800 BC.

Beneficial Results from Massage

- To get good results it is important that the massage should be given in a comfortable environment. Select a warm, calm place with dim lights.

- Always lie on a firm, padded surface to relax the back and the stomach. Always place a cushion under the knees to reduce the arch of the lower back. Place a small cushion or folded towel under the head to raise it about one to three inches.
- In case of giving a soothing massage, use a bed which can leave you relaxed and sleepy.
- Keep your back straight throughout the massage and use the weight of the body to give rhythm and depth to the massage.
- Keep your feet wide apart during massage and bend the knees so that you can lean into the strokes. In case you are working on the floor, kneel with your knees apart.
- Never stay in one position for a long while massaging.
- Wear loose fitting, washable clothes during massage. Avoid wearing shoes; wear flat shoes or be bare-footed.
- Remove all ornaments from the body before giving the massage, as they may cause scratches on the skin while giving massage.
- When massaging the back, put a small cushion or rolled towel under the ankles.
- For a relaxing massage put a cushion under the waist and put another cushion under the shoulder.
- Remember, a firm, brisk massage is invigorating whereas slow, steady massage strokes lead to sleep. Do not repeat the same massage twice.

How to Keep Hands Supple?

The following exercises keep hands supple:

- Hold a rubber ball in one hand and squeeze. Relax the fingers and repeat several times. Follow this exercise on other hand.
- Rotate and stretch each finger and the thumb in each direction. Then pull it gently with the other hand.

- Press and hold the fingers against each other. Do not touch the palms.

Massage Techniques

- A rhythmic massage sends waves of relaxation throughout the body.
- If you feel pain or uncomfortable during massage, inform the masseur.
- Mould your hands to the contours of the body.
- Vary pressure from very light to very strong.
- Massage lightly over the bony areas and firmly over the muscles.
- Do not apply heavy pressure when massaging.
- Avoid talking while massaging. Concentrate only on massage.
- Be totally relaxed when giving a massage.
- Do not worry if your initial massage movements seem clumsy. Practice makes one perfect.

Do not massage if you are suffering from:

- An infection, a contagious disease of the skin.
- High temperature.
- A skin infection, bruises or acute inflammation. An inflammatory condition such as thrombosis or phlebitis.
- Serious inflammatory cases of the joints and in tubercular joints.
- In case of infectious diseases like diphtheria and gonorrhea, which cause formation of pus. Massage may spread the pus to the entire system.

Massage should be done for a few minutes. Sprains and bruises can be cured by massage. In these cases, affected parts should first be bathed with hot water thoroughly. Gentle stroking and kneading is recommended on and around the injured tissues. Fractures can also be treated with massage. Muscles constitute one-half of the weight of the human body and are capable of holding half the blood supply. It becomes all the more important that muscles be kept nourished.

Massage can provide additional nourishment and strength to the tissues.

Massage Movements

Tapping, stroking and vibrating help the muscle develop contractile power. Muscle massage can be done by effleurage and kneading movement, followed by tapotement. Later, active and passive movements are given.

Effect of massage movements: Kneading and percussion strokes cause muscles to contract and become stronger. Deep circular kneading and vibration strokes loosen the muscles. Kneading under and round the muscles breaks adhesions. Massage benefits many nerve problems. In case of acute inflammation of the nerves, massage should be done carefully by light and gentle strokes. Do not apply deep pressure on swollen nerves; it can increase inflammation. All that is needed is just a gentle tapotement or beating of the nerve. Nerve compression is recommended for soothing nerves.

Spinal nerve compression is extremely beneficial in case of insomnia (loss of sleep). It is done with the palms; the vibration of the fingers stimulates spinal nerves. Abdominal massage is beneficial in constipation and stimulates peristalsis of the small intestines, tones up muscles of the abdominal walls. Abdominal massage should not be done in case of the following:

- Inflammation of the uterus, bladder, ovaries and fallopian tubes.
- When suffering from stone in kidney or gall bladder.
- Ulcer of the stomach and intestines.
- In case of pregnancy.
- After taking a heavy meal.

To do abdominal massage, the bladder should be emptied before a massage. The patient is made to lie on the back with knees drawn up to enable the abdominal wall to relax. The masseur should stand on the right side of the patient putting deep and firm pressure with the hands and fingertips.

Chest massage is helpful in many ways. It strengthens the chest muscles, increases circulation and tones up the nerves system of the chest, heart and lungs. It is especially recommended in case of weak lungs, palpitation and organic heart disorders. Chest massage helps to develop bust and mammary glands. In this case, the patient is made to lie on the back with arms at the sides. The masseur starts manipulating the chest with both hands on each side of the breastbone. This massage stimulates the nerves and helps circulation for treating backache, rheumatic afflictions of the back muscles and for soothing the nervous system.

The Theory of Massage Movements

Massage is a method of manipulating the soft tissue of the body. There are five classical massage movements as below:

- **Effluerage:** A stroking movement using the palms of hands or as a large part of the palm that can fit the area that is being worked out. It is used to start or end a massage or as a linking movement between massage. The movement must be flowing and rhythmically with a constant pressure following the venous flow of blood back to the heart. This movement has the following effects:
  1. Aids relaxation.
  2. Warms skin tissues.
  3. Increase blood circulation.
- **Petrissage:** This movement involves lifting the soft tissue away from the underlying structures. Use palm of hands, pads of fingers or thumbs (such as kneading, wringing and skin rolling). It has the following effects:
  1. Softens and relaxes hard contracted muscles.
  2. Eliminates fatigue.
  3. Stimulates sensory nerves.
  4. Increases blood circulation and lymph circulation.
  5. Helps to tone and strengthen muscles.
- **Tapotement:** Also known as percussion movement, which involves striking the skin surface with alternate hands, the wrist has to be loose and mobile in order to

produce a light springy movement (such as cupping, pounding, pinching and hacking). It has the following effects:

1. Increases blood circulation thereby producing erythema.
2. Strengthen and tone the muscles.
3. Stimulate sensory nerves.
4. Increases lymph circulation.
5. Redistribute fatty tissues.

- **Friction:** Small circular movements produced by the pads of the fingers or thumbs to exert pressure. It has the following effects:

1. Break down nodules and fibrous adhesion.
2. Increases blood and lymph circulation.

- **Vibration:** A fine trembling movement using pads of finger and thumb and palms of the hands. This movement can be static or in running form. The movement is always given along a nerve path. It has the following effects:

1. Stimulates the nerves.
2. Loosen scar tissues and stretch adhesion.
3. Relieves pain.

Basic Techniques of Massage

Once you have learnt a few basic movements, you can give a complete body massage. Most of the massage movements have simple variations as below:

- **Stroking:** This rhythmic, flowing movement is very common. Slow movement applied by the palms and fingertips of both hands are calming, while brisk movements are stimulating. Stroking has the following benefits:

1. Improves circulation.
2. Relaxes tense muscles.
3. Soothes jangled nerves.

- **Fan stroking:** It is the simplest type of stroking used on almost all areas of the body. Start with gliding both hands side by side applying a steady, even pressure, to mould the hands to the shape of the body so that the stroke covers the whole body. When stroking the back abdomen, squeeze in slightly at the waist. Avoid dragging the skin and keep hands relaxed. The benefits are similar to those in case of stroking technique as described above.
- **Circle stroking:** Massage in circles or in wide curves pressing firmly on the upward and outward stroke. Place both hands on one side of the body about six inches apart. One hand should do a whole circle and another half circle.
- **Cat stroking:** It is a soothing, soporific movement in which stroke slowly down the body, one hand following other. Do not exert heavy pressure, the hands should barely touch the skin.
- **Thumb stroking:** It is performed with thumbs applying slight pressure firmly upwards with one thumb following the other.
- **Kneading:** This movement is applied on the shoulders, thighs and fleshy areas of the body with slow and deep or fast and stimulating movements. Make sure to use plenty of oil. It has the following benefits:

  1. Relaxes tense muscles.
  2. Improves circulation.
  3. Brings fresh blood and nutrients in the nerves.
  4. Eliminates waste products.

- **Basic kneading movement:** Place hands flat on the skin with fingers and palm pressing down. Grasp the flesh between the fingers and thumbs, and glide towards the other hand. Now release the flesh and grasp with the other hand. Rhythmically squeeze and release flesh with alternative hands.

- **Wringing:** A deeper and more stimulating movement as if wringing out a towel. Pull flesh up with one hand and across towards the other hand pressing deeply with the thumb.
- **Light kneading:** This movement is applied over less fleshy area, such as shoulders and upper arms. Knead lightly, lift and squeeze the flesh between the thumb and fingers. Glide towards the other hand. Squeeze the flesh between thumb and fingers of other hand.
- **Pressure:** This movement releases tension in the muscles and is very relaxing when deep, direct pressure is applied gradually and steadily. Use little oil. This movement is useful for massaging spine and area around the shoulder. Make sure that your thumb-nails do not graze the skin.
- **Static pressure:** Place pads of thumbs on the skin and press for a few seconds. Make small, penetrating circular movements. Release and repeat movement in adjoining area of the skin.
- **Knuckling:** Give small circling strokes. Curl the hand into loose fists with the middle section of the fingers. This movement is very useful for massaging shoulders, chest, palms and soles.
- **Percussion:** A brisk, bouncy movement usually applied on fleshy, muscular areas. Do not apply movement on bony areas, broken veins and bruises. Use this movement at the end of the massage. This movement has the following benefits:
  1. Improves circulation.
  2. Has calming effect and stimulates the nerves.
- **Cradling:** This is a warming, comforting movement with both hands relaxed.
- **Criss-cross movement:** Glide both hands with fingers facing away across the skin.
- **Cat stroking:** This smooth, continuous stroke calms the nerves leaving a soporific effect.

Specialized Massage Movements

- **Therapeutic massage:** Ideal for the treatment of sensitive areas affected by muscular tension, stress and fatigue.
- **Sports massage:** A 50-minute massage treatment done before or after the sports activities to maximize performance potential, reduce muscle fatigue and elimination of toxins.
- **Anti-cellular massage:** Massage movement that works on areas with highest concentration of cellulite. It dissolves the body fat. For excellent results, it should be followed with a steam bath (sauna bath) and completed with shower treatment.
- **Lymphatic massage:** A technique that helps to detoxify the skin of body and drains toxins. It helps to prevent premature ageing.
- **Ultrasonic massage:** It works through an electric device and is very effective for a dull and sallow skin. The massage improves blood circulation, activates sebaceous glands, improve a dry skin and an effective massage treatment in deep penetration of the skin.
- **Suction massage:** It is performed by the portable compressor, which sucks out the infection, bacteria, dirt and dust accumulating on the skin and in skin pores, controls sebum and improves blood circulation.
- **Thai massage:** This traditional massage movement stimulates the flow of energy and the balance is restored on the body - physically, emotionally, mentally and spiritually. This massage therapy ensures several benefits such as release strength, increase energy, give flexibility to the body, provide deep relaxation pressure, improve neurological functions, help stress reduction, promote circulation of blood, restore metabolic balance, promote inner peace and a quiet mind, assist alignment and postural integrity of the body, strengthen inner organs, help homeostasis

balance and harmony and is most suitable for post natal mothers.

- **Japanese massage system:** It is also called Shiatsu. According to this system of massage, the human body has numerous points of energy, which can be described as energy points. By pressing these points, the energy level in the body increases. By giving proper and regular energy on these points, we can regain lost energy, which not only improves the mental health and body metabolism but can also treat physical disharmony simultaneously. This system of massage has also been described in some other chapter in this book.
- **Chinese massage movements:** This massage movement plays an important role to energize and balance the body and mind. It helps to relieve pain, discomfort and many physiological imbalances.
- **Slow massage:** It is done by hitting and vibrating the skin lightly with soft fleshy fingers. In this process, start massaging at slow speed from the neck and gradually increase the speed as it move upward. Stroking gives rest to the nerves and vibrations by fingers, which are useful for subduing pain caused by massaging.
- **Fast massage:** The front halves of both the palms move in circular motion upward, which help in removing wrinkles on the skin.
- **Massage by pinching:** The skin to be massaged is held between the thumb and fingers as in pincers. It cures jaw wrinkles and helps in removing double chin.
- **Pressure massage:** It is applied with fleshy fingertips. This is very effective for removing pouches under the eyes.
- **Massage for pregnant women:** Careful, smooth and gentle massage movements should be applied, which benefit a woman during pregnancy. Do not forget to consult a doctor before applying massage to an

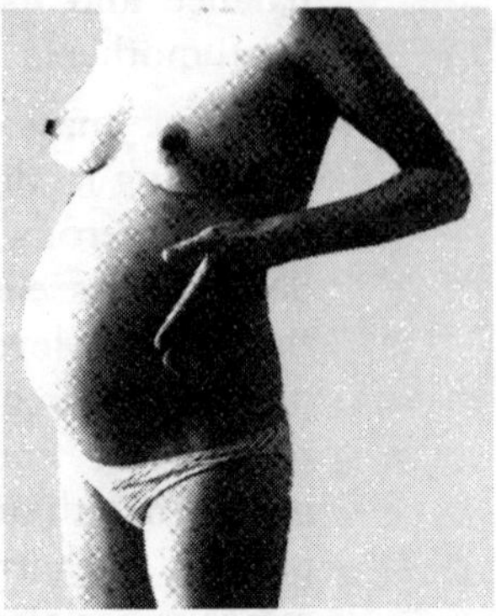

expectant woman. Massage helps alleviate many complications such a tension, backache, insomnia (sleeplessness) and fatty deposits on the body. A pregnant woman should avoid a deep pressure and percussion movements. A careful massage before conception helps to increase the fertility, and three months before the delivery makes labour painless.

You may use all types of movement recommended for abdomen, back, shoulder, leg and feet massage in gentle and very light movements. Use cushion under the shoulder, lower back and knees to reduce curves and discomfort while massaging. Massage done by the trained masseuse makes childbirth easier. Lower back and shoulders are the areas, which relieve tension when massaging. For a back massage, a pregnant woman should lie on her side or sit on a chair, facing towards the back of chair.

Effleurage is a light, rhythmic, stroking massage of the abdomen, back or thighs. It can help with relaxation and pain relief when done on bare skin. Some women prefer an extremely light, even tricky stroking, while others find a firmer touch more soothing. As you and your partner prepare for labour, try varying the pressure and rhythm of effleurage until you find the most appealing stroke. Then practice it as part of your labour preparation. Effleurage over the lower abdomen, following the lower curve of the uterus is most popular. Some people think of it as stroking baby's head. Others like to stroke the abdomen in circles with both hands.

Many women use effleurage during contractions in labour. Keep the massage rhythmic, even timing it with the slow breathing. When finding that the skin is becoming extra sensitive as the contraction intensify, try effleurage in a different area or discontinue it. Other types of massage such as firm stroking or kneading are soothing and relaxing both during pregnancy and during labour. Such massage of the face, neck, shoulders, back, thighs, feet and hands can be very comforting. Work together massaging these different areas and find out how and where massage is most helpful and plan to use it in labour.

Another helpful form of massage for labour is known as counter-pressure used over the lower back during contractions. This type of massage is especially helpful for backache during contractions. Simply press with fist or the heel of the hand on the spot in your low back or sacrum. Press with considerable force, holding hipbone with other hand. The exact spot for applying pressure varies from woman to woman and found most helpful and relaxing.

The following massage movements are beneficial for a pregnant woman:

1. Apply gentle stroking firstly with one hand, then with both hands, one following the other clockwise on the abdomen.
2. Stroke softly on the side of the waist upwards with one hand after the other till both hands reach the navel. Now gently glide the hands towards the abdomen downward, and then to the sides to complete the stroke.
3. Cup your hands over the navel for a few seconds till you feel the heat. Slowly remove hands.
4. Leg massage, too, is very beneficial for pregnant women. It soothes, relaxes and relieves swelling and pain in legs, cures varicose veins and leg cramps usually faced by expectant mothers.
5. The best remedy is to sleep with the legs slightly raised above the level of head, which relieves swelling in the legs.
6. Massage purifies and corrects drainage system of the body, melts fat deposits, calms the nerves, drains waste products and toxins and cures many

skin disorders like eczema, acne, dermatitis etc. related with pregnancy.

7. Light stroking movements may be applied on the mid back just above the waist, at the base of spine and between the shoulder blades on the back of an expecting mother.
8. Press firmly applying circular pressure with your thumbs on the hips and buttocks to relieve lower back pain and melt fat deposits on the hips and thighs.
9. Foot massage pressing few shiatsu points can relieve pain during labour and help speedy delivery. Stroke the sole of the feet firmly with the heel of your hand. Apply deep pressure with thumbs in the centre of the sole to the heel of the feet, which reduce labour pains.

- **Massage after the childbirth:** A deep massage to abdomen for 40 days after the delivery of baby energizes the mother, cures body aches and brings uterus back to its original position. The following abdominal massage movements should be applied:
  1. Stroke abdomen in all directions. Knead firmly on hips and gently across the abdomen.
  2. Stroke clockwise in large circles on the abdomen applying gentle pressure.
  3. Stroke slowly up the abdomen starting at the pubic bone and pressing with heels of hands.
  4. Stroke slowly on the lower abdomen starting from the pubic bone to the navel.
  5. Finally cup your hands over the navel and hold for few seconds until you feel heat accumulating beneath the hands. Now lift hands slowly.

The Healing Power of Massage

- **The lymph drainage:** The lymphatic system acts as a purifying and drainage system and plays an important part in fighting infection and developing immunity.

There are lymph vessels and nodes throughout the body. The nodes are present in the neck, armpits, groin, behind the knees and on the inside of the elbows. Massage can energize the lymph throughout the body, thus eliminating waste and strengthening the immune system.

- **Fight stress:** A stressed mind becomes calm, quiet, peaceful and refreshed after a massage. High blood pressure and heart diseases are related to stress. Disorders such as cancer, rheumatism, headaches, backache, acne, infertility and infectious skin diseases are more likely to develop when resistance is low. Massage helps to reduce physical as well as emotional stress and relax taut muscles, enabling the body and mind to relax.
- **Insomnia relief:** In case of insomnia, general massage at bedtime promotes sleep and complete relaxation of the body. Keep all your movements smooth, rhythmic, and hypnotic. Massage the back, abdomen and feet using rhythmic stroking movements, which leads to good sleep. Pressing certain points induces uninterrupted sleep.
    1. Press between eyebrows with your thumb and hold pressure for 10-15 seconds, then release.
    2. Press inside of your wrist below the little finger with your thumb. Hold for 10-15 seconds. Now repeat on the other wrist.
    3. Press anklebone on the inside of your ankle. Rest your little finger on the bony prominence and the index finger behind the shinbone. Press your thumb for ten seconds on each ankle.

Massage with Aromatic Oils

It is very useful for the skin, vigour and vitality. Mostly people with excessive oily skin use talcum powder for massage. Use a light vegetable oil for massage. Do not pour the oil directly on to the body. Pour about a teaspoon of oil into the palm, then rub your hands together to warm them slightly and massage. Essential oils blended with massage oil add new dimension to massage and impart a feeling of luxury to the massage. The perfume in the oil helps to relax or refresh. Essential oils have different properties. Some of them are anti-bacterial. Others have antiseptic or anti-inflammatory properties.

Aromatherapy: Aromatherapy is fast gaining popularity as an alternative or holistic medicine for the balance of body, mind and spirit. Derived from the ancient practice of using natural plant essence to soothe nerves and promote health, this therapy was initially primarily used to adorn bodies. The therapy works on the mind through the pores of the skin. The plant extracts enter the body through inhalation or massage. Self-practice of aromatherapy without full know how is not advisable as concentrated oils are very strong and can have diverse effects. Each aroma used must be acceptable to the body for positive effects.

Aroma Massage on Reflex Points

Massage the reflex points on the body with small, stationary, circular movements applying pressure about three seconds at each point as below, which helps to slim, tone, energize and relax the body:

- On the sole of foot.
- Behind the ankle bone.
- Ball of the foot.
- On the back of waistline.
- On the back above waistline.
- On the back on either side of vertebrae.
- On the front, three inches below the navel.
- On one inch either side of the navel.
- On four inches above the navel.
- At the lower cheekbone on both sides.
- On either side of nose.
- The hollow below the ears.

Refreshing Massage

- Rest your forearms on the shoulders. This will reduce tension.
- Stroke firmly up the back on either side of the spine.
- Knead the muscles across the top of the shoulders with both hands squeezing.

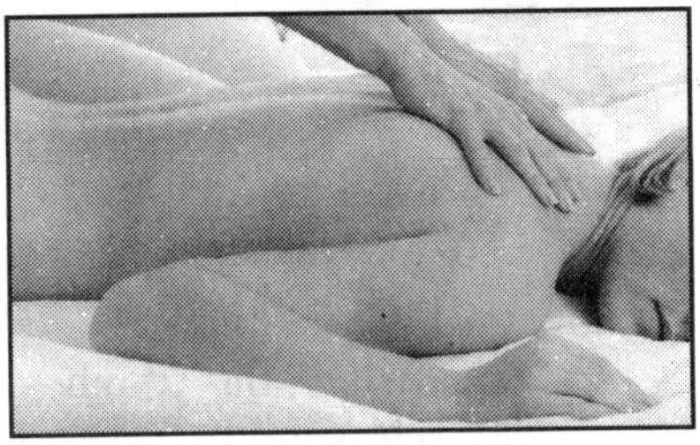

- Calm the shoulder muscle pressing gently to drain out tension.
- Place thumbs on either side of the spine. Hold the exert pressure for few seconds, followed by stroking the upper and lower back and shoulder blades.
- Now massage the back of the neck at the base of the skull with the right hand applying circular pressure, supporting the head with the left hand.
- Use both hands to massage the complete head including the area around the ears, on the temples and forehead.
- Rub your hair briskly back and forth with your fingertips. This relieves tension.
- Stimulate the shoulders and upper back with the sides of the hands. Keep hands relaxed. Avoid kidney and spinal area.
- Soothe the whole back with rhythmic massage movements followed by the feather stroke.

A Self-massage

- **Self-massage of legs and thighs:** Legs massage relieves aching, stimulates circulation of blood and the lymphatic system. The following steps are advised for a self-leg massage:

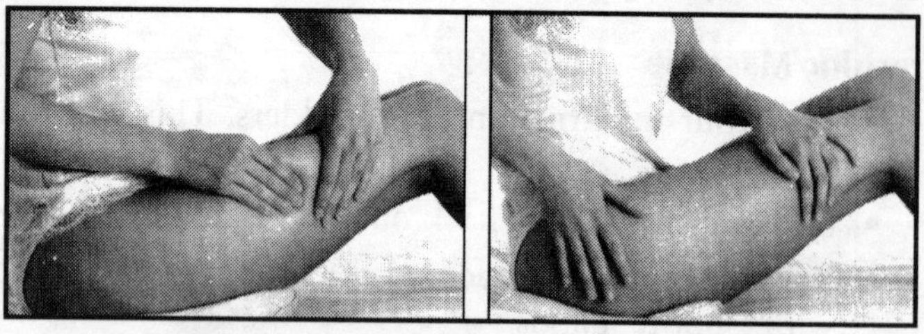

1. Stroke the whole leg from ankle to thigh with one hand on each leg beginning at the foot, up the calf, over the knee and up to the top of thigh molding your hands to the shape of your legs and thighs.
2. Knead the thighs rhythmically, squeezing and releasing the flesh. Now soothe from the knee with one hand following the other, which helps to improve the shape and texture.
3. Pummel the thighs with loosely clenched fists of your hands, which bring blood to the surface and relieve stiffness in the nerves. Remember, to stroke your knees softly with circular pressure massage with your fingertips.
4. Finally knead the calf muscles, squeezing with both hands exerting the bone.

- **Abdomen self-massage:** Abdomen and hip massage provides comfort to the whole body. Work the following steps:

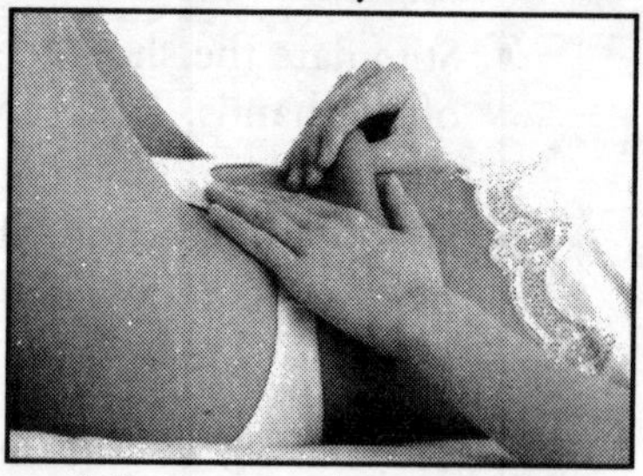

1. Lie down to massage yourself with your knees bent up. Stroke your abdomen clockwise with both hands open. Knead all over your abdomen with your fingers and thumb. Then knead your hips and bottom.
2. Cup your hands over your navel until you feel the heat, then lift slowly.

3. Pummel your hips and bottom vigorously with loosely clenched fists. This will leave you feeling refreshed and energized.

- **Arms self-massage:** Arm massage helps to dissolve tension in the arms and shoulders besides refreshing and soothing the nerves. Work the following steps:

1. Stroke from wrist to shoulders and glide back.

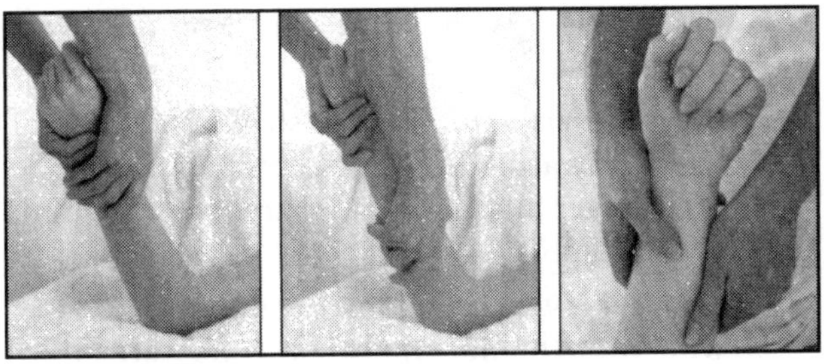

2. Knead the upper arm squeezing and releasing the fleshy area.
3. Apply circular pressure on your forearm with your thumbs.
4. Pat your arm to stimulate the circulation in the muscles.
5. Finish the massage stroking your whole arm.

- **Self-feet and hand massage:** It is very easy to massage your feet and hands. Foot problems lead to bad posture, backache and weariness. Tired hands lead to tension. You can relieve tiring, exhaustion and tension by regular feet and hand massage with the help of following massage movements:

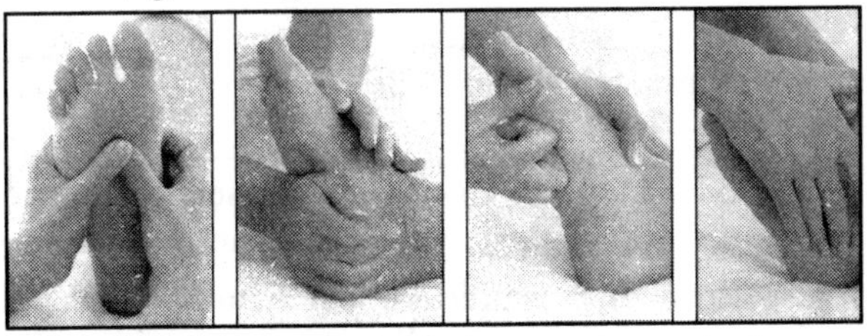

1. Start massaging under the sole and then stroke smoothly from toe to your ankles and back to the

toes. Squeeze each toe firmly followed by stretching.

2. Press the centre of the sole with thumbs giving circular motion around on the ball of the feet.
3. Do knuckling movements all over the sole in circular movements.
4. Hack the sole with the ends of your hand. Stroke the ankles with your fingertips. Reverse all movements.
5. For self-massaging hands, stroke the back of your hands towards the wrist gently and back. Squeeze each finger and apply pressure over the joints with your thumb.
6. Stroke between tendons on the back of the hand with your thumb. Apply static pressure all over the palm with your thumb.
7. Finish the massage by stroking the palm with fingers.

- **Neck and chin self-massage:** The following movements stimulate the circulation of neck muscles and prevent development of double chin:

1. Stroke from the collarbone to chin using back of your hands to massage one side, one hand following the other. Now repeat this movement to the other side.
2. Pinch along your jaw line with thumbs and knuckles of your fingers, starting from chin to the ears without stretching.
3. Slap gently under the chin with your hands alternately. This will stimulate the muscles under the chin.
4. Now stroke from the corners of your mouth towards the ears with one hand on each cheek.
5. Press the temples under your fingers, clenching your teeth to stimulate the jaw muscles.

- **Self eye massage:** To dissolve lines and wrinkles under the eyes the following massage movements should be tried:
  1. Stroke gently with middle finger in a circle round your eyes, working from the bridge of your nose over your eyebrows pressing temples.
  2. Pinch along your eyebrows from the centre to the temples.
  3. With your thumbs and index finger press the bone under the eyebrows at the bridge of the nose.

How to Practice Shiatsu?

Shiatsu therapy, also known as acupressure, is used to treat disorders by pressing various pressure points on the skin. There are nearly 600 shiatsu points in the human body and few of them are very important, which we shall discuss here. Pressure points produce energy that flows in the body and cures diseases.

Shiatsu treatments are given on the floor. Lie face down on a towel. Keep both hands moving rhythmically along the meridians from one point to the other, pressing each point from three to five seconds. When breathing, run down either side of the spine. It takes about 45 to 60 minutes to treat the whole body, which improves the circulation and induces relaxation. The following steps are carried out to practice shiatsu:

- Press down either side of the spine.
- Use the heels of the hands, then repeat with the thumbs.
- Press down the buttocks and the back of the legs, keeping light pressure over the knees.
- Now turn the direction, squeeze down arms, pressing on the points on the arms and hands.
- Apply pressure down on the front of the legs.
- Press gently on the abdomen, working clockwise in large circles.

- Kneel and press on all the points.
- Work from the centre of the chest outwards, pressing in lines between the ribs.

Shiatsu points on the face are following:

• Centre of hairline to the crown of head	Relieves headache.
• On the centre of eyebrow	Relieves headache/migraine
• On top edge of cheek bone	Relieves headache/migraine
• Between the nose and upper lip	Helps weight reduction.
• Between the eyebrows	Relieves headache/migraine
• Inside corners of eyes	Relieves tired eyes.
• Below end of eyebrows	Relieves headache/migraine.
• Grooves at the side of nose	Relieves facial tension, sinus, toothache and clears nasal congestion.

Important pressure (shiatsu) points on the front of body are the following:

1. Groove between ribs	Relieves cough and chest pain.
2. Deltoid muscles	Eases tension.
3. Below the elbow dispels nervousness.	Soothes hand and arm muscles.
4. Below knees	Alleviates body pain and restore energy.
5. Centre of abdomen	Alleviates menstrual problems, Cures constipation.
6. Between thumb and finger	Dispel pain and headache (Pregnant women should avoid).
7. Outer thighs below waist	Stimulates circulation and relaxes tired legs and body.

8. Above inside ankle	Eases menstrual pain and labour problems.

Important pressure points on the back of body are following:

1. Crown of head	Dispel headache, backache and fatigue.
2. Base of skull on neck	Relieve headache, sinus and stiff neck.
3. Chin	Dispel headache, cold and sinus problem.
4. On the sacrum	Relieve lower back and menstrual pain.
5. Side muscles	Strengthen heart and lungs, digestion and strengthen reproductive sex organs.
6. Hip	Relieve menstruation pain and backache.
7. Middle of calf muscle	Relieve back pain and tired legs.
8. Ankles	Remove stomach pain and relaxes body.
9. Centre of palms	Stimulates energy and remove nervousness.
10. Upper back	Relieves headache and stiff shoulder.
11. On the buttock	Reduce tension in lower back.
12. Centre of shoulder blade	Reduce stiffness of shoulders.
13. Outside/inside of ankles	Relieve menstrual pain.

Keep in mind the following points when applying pressure on shiatsu points:

- Let the pressure come from shoulders.
- Keep your arms straight when applying pressure.

- Press with the balls of your thumb.
- Increase pressure steadily and evenly on the shiatsu points by leaning your body weight on hands.
- Keep your knees apart to give a steady base when applying pressure.
- Swing your hips forward to apply gradual pressure.
- Rest your fingers lightly when applying pressure on the back.
- Apply pressure lightly, steadily and evenly on delicate areas such as abdomen and the face.

How to Loose Weight by Massage?

The following massage steps are advised for weight loss:

- Squeeze either side of the wrist above the wrist bone.
- Press on the hollow inside of the ankles just behind the bony prominence.
- Press at the middle of the groove between the nose and upper lip.

To fight overweight, pay attention on the fleshiest areas of the body such as abdomen, thighs and buttocks using stimulating movements such as kneading and pummeling. Vigorous massage helps in slimming. Remember, massage alone without regular exercise and control over the diet cannot reduce weight or break down fat. Massage tones the skin, soothes the body, produce energy by stimulating the circulation. Weight watchers should concentrate on self-massage of the following fleshiest areas:

- **Abdomen:** Lie on your back and knead abdomen.
- **Hips:** Roll on one side, knead and pummel both hips.
- **Thighs:** Sit up and knead thighs from knee up to the hips vigorously.
- **Buttocks:** Pummel fast over thighs up to the buttocks.

3

Massage Techniques

Massage Treatment for Weight Loss

Massage treatment is very useful to melt extra fat from the body, especially in women after the age of 50, during pregnancy and after childbirth. Practice the following steps:

- Squeeze either side of the wrist above the wrist bone.
- Press on the hollow inside the ankles just behind the bony prominence.
- Press in the middle of the groove between nose and upper lip.

To fight overweight, pay attention on the fleshiest areas of the body such as abdomen, thighs and buttocks using stimulating movements such as kneading and pummeling. Vigorous massage helps in slimming. Remember massage alone without regular exercise and control over the diet cannot reduce weight or break down fat. Massage tones the skin, soothes the body, produces energy by stimulating the circulation. Weight watchers should concentrate on self-body massage of the following fleshiest areas:

- **Abdomen:** Lie on your back and knead abdomen thoroughly.
- **Hips:** Roll on to one side; knead and pummel both hips.
- **Thighs:** Sit up and knead thighs from knee up to the hips vigorously.
- **Buttocks:** Pummel fast over thighs up to the buttock.

Massage for Brides before Marriage

In case of a heavy figure with fat deposits over abdomen, hips, thighs and buttocks a proper daily massage is essential at the time of bath two to three weeks before marriage. Massage with a massaging cream has miraculous effect on the skin. A special recipe (paste) for brides to be used daily can be prepared by mixing the following ingredients and rubbing it thoroughly to stimulate the skin:

Dried ground lemon peel	1 tablespoon
Almond powder	½ tablespoon
Wheat-germ flour	4 tablespoons
Ground thyme	1 tablespoon
Almond oil	3-4 drops
Jasmine oil	3-4 drops
Salt	a pinch

Rub on the body thoroughly for 30 minutes before taking bath.

Massage for Expectant Mothers

Massage helps alleviate many complications during period of pregnancy and after delivery of baby, which include mental tension, backache, insomnia, lines and wrinkles on abdomen and fatty deposits on the body. Avoid deep pressure and percussion. A careful massage is definitely beneficial during pregnancy and before conception to increase the fertility of a woman. Use all stroking techniques for massaging abdomen, back, shoulders, legs and foot massage ensuring very light and gentle strokes. Massage done by a trained masseuse makes childbirth easier. Lower back and shoulders are the areas to concentrate for relieving tension while massaging. The various massage movements for a pregnant woman include gentle stroke on the abdomen with hands, one following the other clockwise. Stroke softly on the sides of the stomach upwards with hands, one following the other till hands reach the navel. Then glide hands gently towards abdomen. Cup your hands over the navel for few seconds until you feel the heat, then lift hands slowly. A regular abdomen massage makes child delivery easy and painless.

Leg massage during pregnancy: is especially beneficial, soothing, relaxing, relieving swelling and pain in legs. Varicose veins or cramps in the leg muscle are common problems often faced by expectant women. Such women should always sleep with legs and feet slightly raised above the level of head. This sleeping posture relieves swollen legs by aiding manual lymph drainage. This lymphatic pumping system drains off the waste products from the body and ensure healthy environment in the body cells by pumping out waste products and bacteria from the blood and circulate purified blood in the body. Besides slimming and eliminating the waste from the body, backache, morning sickness the massage helps in strengthening the immune system curing many skin disorders like acne, eczema, dermatitis and skin inflammation.

Arms and back massage during pregnancy: Arm massage during this period leaves soothing effect on the body when restrictions of abdomen massage are advised for expectant mothers. Backache and morning sickness are the common complaints during pregnancy, which can be relieved to a great extent with back massage. Avoid deep pressure to the lower back. Back pain can be alleviated with plenty of smooth and flowing stroking movements on the mid back just above the waist at the base of spine and between shoulder blades. Press firmly by applying circular pressure with your thumb on the hips and buttocks.

Massage After Childbirth

Massage to abdomen for minimum 40 days after the delivery of baby energizes the mother, cures body aches, sheds extra flesh and brings uterus to the original position prior to delivery. To give an abdomen massage to women after childbirth the following steps should be applied:

- Stroke the abdomen in all directions.
- Knead firmly on hips, gently across the abdomen.
- Stroke clockwise in large circles on the abdomen applying gentle pressure.

- Stroke slowly up on the lower abdomen starting from the pubic bone to the navel.
- Cup hands over the navel for few seconds until you feel heat under the hands. Then lift hands slowly.

How to Massage the Face?

- Blend a little cleansing cream with the fingers to soften it. Using both hands apply cream over the face applying following massage movements:
- Start at the chin and with a sweeping movement slide to end of jaw.
- Continue from base of nose to temple, along the side of nose, between the brows, and across forehead to temples.

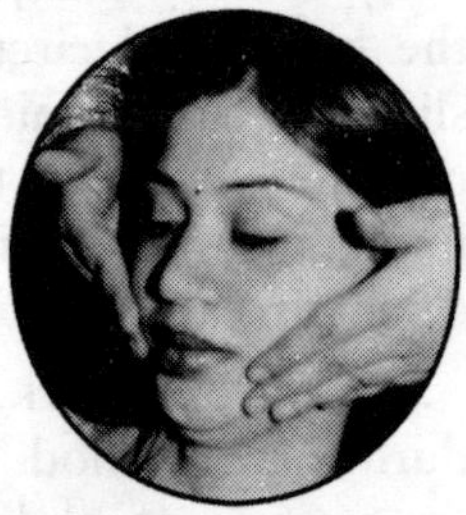

- Now take additional cream, blend it, smooth down the neck, chest and back.
- Next start massaging at the centre of forehead, move lightly around eyes, then towards temples and back to the centre of the forehead.
- Slide down from nose to upper lip, smooth to temples and forehead, then move lightly down to chin and finally slide up towards jaw line, temples and forehead.
- Remove cream with cleansing tissues or warm moist towel.
- Emollient cream selected according to skin type should be applied in the same manner as indicated above.
- Use lanolin or hormone cream for a dry skin and cold cream for an oily skin.
- For neck, face, shoulder and chest, apply emollient cream.
- Apply eye cream under the eyes gently with fingertips.

- Use muscle oil around the neck.
- For massaging face apply a massage cream giving manipulations using slightly cupped hands and fingers. Start massage under the lower lip with two fingers. Repeat process several times. Pinch gently along the jaw line, working outward ears.

Massage is one of the easiest ways for attaining and maintaining health, youth, vigour, beauty, melting extra fat and relive tension and stress. According to expert's advice, when couples touch each other and embrace, can prevent physical and mental illness. It improves circulation, relax muscles, aids digestion by stimulating the lymphatic system, eliminates waste products, provides energy, refreshes and revitalize body. The word massage has been derived from the Arabic word 'Masah', which means the magic of hands.

Important tips for massage are the following:

- Early morning massage has a miraculous effect on the various organs. To get beneficial results, it is important that massage is given in a comfortable environment. Choose a warm, peaceful place with dim lights.
- Always lie on a firm, padded surface to relax the back and the stomach. Place a cushion under the knees to reduce the arch of the lower back and place a small cushion or folded towel under the head.
- A hard bed is ideal if you want to give a soothing massage, which can leave you relaxed and sleepy.
- Keep your back straight throughout the massage and use the weight of your body to give rhythm and depth.
- Never stay in one position when massaging.
- Wear loose-fitting washable clothes and be bare-footed.
- Remove ornament before massage, it can cause scratches.
- Support a sway back with a cushion under the waist.

- If you feel pain or an uncomfortable situation during massage, inform the masseur.
- Mould your hands to the contours of the body.
- Vary pressure from very light to very strong. The massage should be lighter over bony areas and firmer over the muscles. Do not apply heavy pressure when massaging.
- Concentrate on the massage. Avoid talking when massaging. Feel totally relaxed for a good massage.
- Do not worry if your initial movements seem clumsy. Practice will make you perfect.

Avoid Massage, if You Suffer from

- An infection or a contagious skin disease.
- High temperature.
- Skin infection, bruises or an acute inflammation.
- An inflammatory condition such as thrombosis or phlebitis.
- Inflammatory cases of joints.
- Infectious diseases like diphtheria and gonorrhea, which cause formation of pus; a massage may spread the pus to entire system.
- During pregnancy without consulting your doctor.

Few Massage Techniques

- **Reflexology massage (75-minute treatment):** Finger pressure is applied to the reflex points of feet to stimulate the related organs of the body and to restore balance and muscular systems.
- **Relaxing massage (50-minute treatment):** It relieves stress, reduces muscle fatigue and improves blood circulation resulting in shedding extra fat deposits.
- **Therapeutic massage:** An ideal massage for toning the muscles, treatment of sensitive areas affected by muscular tension, stress and fatigue.

- **Sports massage (50-minute treatment):** It helps to reduces muscle fatigue and eliminates toxins produced in the muscles during physical exercise.
- **Anti-cellulite massage:** A reductive massage that works in parts with the highest concentrations of cellulite. It generates heat to help dissolve body fat. Excellent results are obtained when it is followed by a sauna session (steam bath) and completed with a shower bath.
- **Lymphatic drainage:** A massage technique, which helps to detoxify the skin of the body. This massage movement helps to drain toxins, prevent fatness and control premature ageing.
- **Shiatsu-massage:** A massage technique in which 'shi' means finger and 'Atsu' means the pressure. In this movement, the fingers, palms and sometimes elbow are used to exercise pressure on few pressure points of the body to stimulate energy. This massage technique reduces stress, alleviates aches, pains, fatigue and fat deposits on the body.
- **Ultrasonic massage therapy:** It helps to provide glow, improve blood circulation, activate sebaceous glands, improve dry dull and sallow skins. It is highly effective massage treatment to slim body especially beneficial in winter season.
- **Suction massage therapy:** It sucks out infection, harmful bacteria, dirt, dust, germs from the upper layer of the epidermis and from the deeper stratum. The benefits of this massage include tightening of the skin, leaving it germs-free, helping to control sebum, improve blood circulation and removes infection.
- **Thai massage:** A massage therapy recognized as an effective mean of reducing stress, pain, muscular and general relaxation, recovery from injury, circulation of blood and lymph and restoration of metabolic balance. Thai massage is a combination of

acupressure, breathing technique, gentle stretches and beautiful postures.

- **Under eye massage:** To dissolve lines and wrinkles under the eyes, following massage movements should be tried:

Stroke gently with middle finger in circle round the eyes. Work from the bridge of your nose out over your eyebrows, pressing the temples. Pinch along the eyebrow from the centre to the temples. Press the bone under the eyebrows at the bridge of the nose with your thumbs and index fingers.

What is Lymphatic Massage?

This massage technique helps in purifying the blood from the heart (on left side) and lymphatic ducts those exist on right side through 18 lymphatic nodes in human body. Lymphatic massage has following advantages:

- The waste products are released from the body.
- Helps fighting bacteria and infections and removes wastage from tissues.
- Improves blood circulation.
- Melts extra fat deposits on the body.
- Relaxes nodes.
- The waste fluids get removed from the veins through urine.
- Excellent for curing acne and skin diseases.

Following precautions are essential during lymphatic massage:

- Lie straight for lymphatic massage.
- Avoid massage if the age is below 16 years.
- Wrongly done massage is harmful; may cause vomiting and headache.
- Massage can be done on every type of skin.
- Remove make-up before massage and cleanse the skin thoroughly.

- The massage movements should be carried by touch therapy (effleurage movement) or with the help of a electrical gadgets.

Body Massage

Massage is a scientific method of giving manipulations to the body by rubbing, pinching, kneading, tapping or stroking with the hands and fingers with the help of various types of massage creams and oils available in market. Body massage has the following benefits:

- Stimulates and smoothen the nerves.
- Relieves body tension.
- Increases circulation of blood.
- Causes muscles contraction.
- Stimulates the action of skin glands.
- Helps to relieve pain in the muscles.
- Softens the skin.
- Calms, relaxes and relieves emotional tension.
- And above all, it alleviates and melts fat.

Precautions when Massaging

- Do not massage over an area where redness, swelling, pus is present.
- Do not break contact with the skin until the massage is finished.
- Always massage towards origin of the muscles.
- Keep fingernail short enough, to avoid scratching the skin.
- Carry out massage rhythmically from the insertion to the origin of muscles.
- Massaging in wrong direction causes muscles and the skin to sag.

Some Don'ts

Massage should not be done in the following conditions:

- Heart diseases.
- High blood pressure.

- Inflamed or swollen joints.
- Glandular swelling.
- Abrasions of the skin.
- A skin disease.
- Broken capillaries.

Some Do's while Massaging

- A firm, sure touch.
- Develop strong flexible hands.
- Self control.
- Quiet temperament.
- Use of psychology.
- Leveled nails to prevent scratching, warm, dry hands.

Baby Massage

Massaging a newly born baby helps to reduce colic pain, constipation, diarrhea, and contraction of muscles. Use gentle strokes and a light vegetable oil for massaging a child, almond oil and sunflower oil are most suitable for massaging babies, since baby oil is not easily absorbed by the baby skin. Here are few tips for baby massage:

- Stroke the baby's forehead from the centre to the sides. Now stroke baby's face from nose to the temples. Press softly for a few seconds and glide down to the chin. Then circle the eyes stroking very gently along the eyebrows and under the eyes.

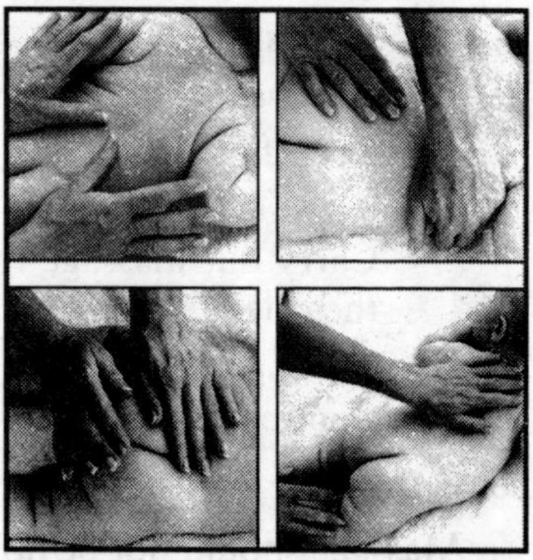

- Stroke from the thighs and glide up to the shoulders. Now massage the sides of the body including the abdomen in criss-cross movement. Finally, massage in clockwise circle round the navel. These soothing massage movements relieve colic pain and stomach aches.

- Turn your baby on his or her front for a back massage. Start from bottom upward at the back, gliding your hands out across the shoulders. Stroke with your thumbs up the back on either side of the spine.
- Now stroke round each buttock and knead gently. Rhythmically pat and pinch your baby's bottom softly. Finish the back massage with the cat stroke and glide your hands smoothly over the back.
- Massaging baby's arms and legs are equally important. Stroke down from the shoulders to the hand, uncurl and squeeze the fingers one by one.
- Stroke legs and finally stroke the feet, and squeeze and rotate each toe.

Child Massage

Smooth, rhythmic stroking of child's tummy round the navel and abdomen in clockwise direction can be very soothing for children. It rids the child of tummy ache and improves digestive system. There is no need to undress the child. Always use light vegetable oil, such as almond or sunflower oil for the massage. Avoid massage after a heavy meal.

Massage Treatments for Curing Body Disorders

Curing varicose veins

Permanently and unevenly dilated veins cause lightness and arching in affected area where blood doesn't flow smoothly in veins developing clots. A very gentle massage in consultation with doctor can be beneficial in relieving the condition. Stroke round the varicose vein, but avoid massaging on the vein, which could dislodge a clot causing harm. Avoid stimulating movement (pummeling and hacking) on varicose veins. However, you can do a massage over varicose vein by gently stroking the area around the vein. Stroke the whole thigh from the knee upwards. Stroke round the knee cap with your thumbs and behind the knee with your fingers, stroking up the leg gently. Now stroke up the calf.

Curing Cramps

If you are prone to cramps during or after exercise, massage will be beneficial in curing it. A cramped muscle lacks proper blood supply. Massage improves circulation of blood. Cramps usually exist in leg, calf or foot.

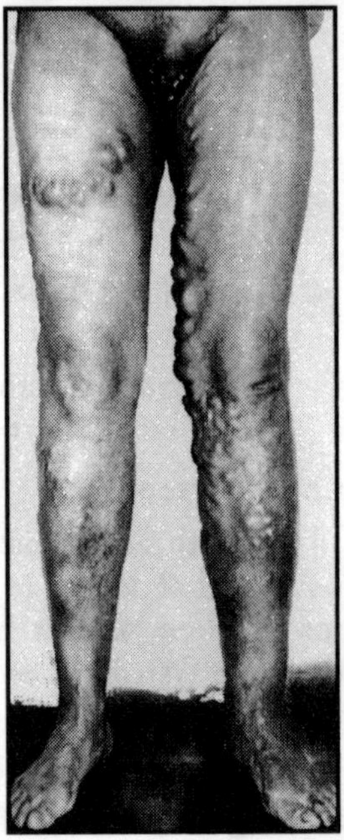

- **Leg cramp:** To soothe cramps in the leg, lie on your back. Raise the affected leg, stroke the back of your thighs, then knead it and finally stroke the affected area.
- **Calf cramp:** To treat cramps in calf, sit with the affected leg straight. Bend your foot up and stretch the calf muscles. Knead the muscle firmly. When you feel the muscle relaxing, soothe it by rhythmically stroking the whole leg.
- **Foot cramp:** Hold your toes and bend them back. Stroke and knead the soles of your feet.

Curing Sprained Ankle and Joints

To reduce swelling and relieving pain, massage sprained ankle and joints for approximately ten minutes several times a day until the injury is healed. To treat, carry the following steps:

- Start stroking up the thigh towards the lymph nodes in the groin.
- Stroke up the sides of the calf to the knees and back to the ankles massaging with your thumbs.

- A sprained wrist or a knee can be treated in the same way. Consult a doctor before the massage. Be careful not to press on any visible vein.

Curing Backache

80 to 90 per cent of backaches are usually caused by painful muscles. Massage is an ideal technique for relieving muscular problems. Muscular pain can be treated by shiatsu therapy applying pressure on certain shiatsu points. Each pressure point is pressed with thumbs for ten seconds. Following are important pressure points on the body to treat aching muscles:

- Press on either side of the spine six inches above the waistline.
- Press at the back of the thighs just under the buttocks.
- Press in the centre of the hollow on the side of the buttock.
- Press in the middle of the back of the thighs.
- Press half way down the thighs.
- Press half way down the back of the calf.

Curing Stomach Ache

- Press at the points two inches below the navel.
- Press in the grooves behind the shin bone two inches below the knee

Curing Sinus Headache and Migraine

For the treatment, the following steps are advised:

- Press the middle of each eyebrow and between the eyebrows.
- Press on the cheekbone below the centre of your eyes.
- Pinch both sides of your hand just below the knuckle at the base of your little finger.

In case you suffer from migraine, following steps help to cure:

- Press between the outer corner of the eye and the eyebrow.

- Press the base of the skull.
- Pinch the web of skin between the thumb and forefinger.

Curing Common cold

There are several shiatsu points on the body that provide quick remedies just by pressing for four to eight seconds.

- Press the skin between the thumb and the forefinger.
- Press at the base of skull on the back.

Curing Painful Menstruation

Squeeze on either side of the ankle just behind the bony prominence and on the inside of the leg three inches above the prominence.

In Case of Lack of Energy and Sex power

- Press just below the ball of the foot on the centre of the sole.
- Squeeze skin at the middle of the palm of the hand.
- Press the groove behind the shinbone, three inches below the knee.

Pre-exercise and After-exercise Massage

Exercising tense muscles can damage them badly. Tense muscles do more work than the required and in the process, consume more oxygen as well as well produce more wastes. Ideally, do a whole body massage with stimulating movements increase blood supply before exercising. During exercise, waste products such as urea, acetic and carbolic acids are released into the muscles and accumulation of these waste cause stiffness and pain. The lymphatic system, however, drains these wastes, but the process is very slow. Massage can speed up the elimination. The following precautions are necessary before or after an exercise:

- Massage firmly towards the heart with gentle stroking towards the lymph nodes.
- Avoid massage directly on an injury. Just work very gently around it, stroking towards the nearest lymph

nodes and kneading gentle above and to the side of the injury.

- Never massage around the open wound.

Shiatsu Therapy

Also known as acupressure therapy, which is used to treat disorders by pressing each pressure point on the body for three to five seconds. There are nearly 600 Shiatsu Points on the human body, which produces energy that flows in the body. It takes about 45 to 60 minutes to treat the whole body. Prominent pressure points exist on either side of the spine, abdomen, centre of the chest, buttocks, back and front of the legs, arms and hands. The following precautions are observed while doing Shiatsu massage.

- Keep arms straight exerting pressure from shoulders.
- Apply pressure with the balls of thumb and fingers.
- Increase pressure steadily and evenly.
- Keep knees apart and swing hips forward to apply gradual pressure.
- Apply pressure lightly, steadily and evenly on abdomen especially in case of pregnant women.
- The lighting should be dimmed. Many people like to hear music while having massage, others enjoy in total peace and quiet and few may like to talk. The best is gentle music that suits most tastes.
- Remove all clothes before massage for better treatment.

Aroma Massage

Essential oils have a therapeutic effect on the body as they are analgesic, antibiotic, anti-fungal, anti-inflammatory, antioxidant, antiseptic, anti-spasmodic, anti-viral, carminative, depurative, digestive, diuretic, expectorant, hepatic, laxative, hypersensitive, sedative, stimulant and toning. Essential oils help to restore balance to the emotions and mind, which are capable to:

- Restore balance to the emotions and mind.
- Soothe nervous tension and worries.

- Melt extra fat.
- Improve concentration and memory.
- Uplift depression and negativity.
- Induce deep relaxation, relieving both physical and mental fatigue.
- Improve circulation to the muscles, thereby inducing inflammation and pain.
- Release neck and shoulder tension and backache.
- Relieve neuralgic arthritis and rheumatic conditions.
- Help sprains, fractures, breaks and heals easily.
- Promote correct posture and help improve mobility.
- Improve the function of every internal organ.
- Improve digestion, assimilation and elimination.
- Relieve constipation.
- Increase the ability of the kidneys to function efficiently.
- Flush the lymphatic system by the mechanical elimination of toxins and waste matter.
- Reduce high blood pressure.
- Help disperse headaches or migraines.
- Stimulate mind and body without any side effect.
- Stimulate the immune system.
- Help relieve suppressed feelings.
- Encourage deep breathing.

4

Face Massage to Tone Muscles

Blend a little cleansing cream with the fingers to soften it. Use both hands when applying cream over the face with the following massage movements:

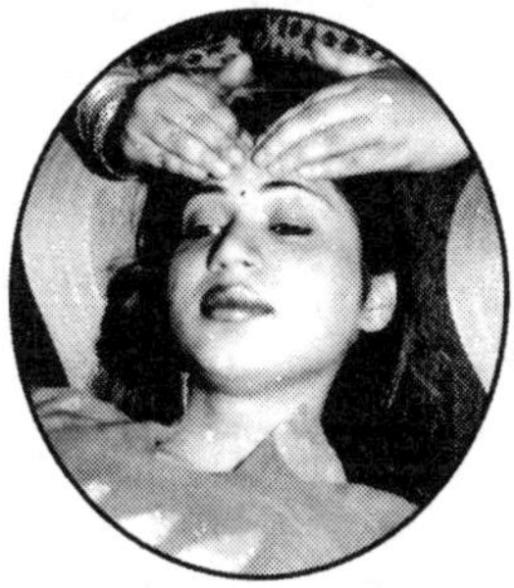

- Start at the chin with a sweeping movement. Slide hand towards the end of jaw.
- Continue massage movement from the base of nose towards the temple, along the side of nose, between the brows, and across forehead to temples.
- Take additional massage cream, blend it, smooth down the neck, chest and back.

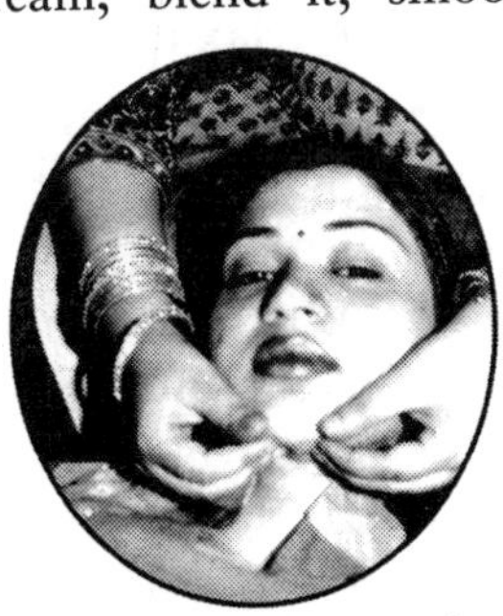

- Now start massaging at the centre of forehead and move lightly around the eyes, towards the temples and back to the centre of forehead.
- Slide hands down from nose towards upper lip. Smooth temples and the

forehead, and move hands lightly down to the chin and finally slide up towards jaw line, temples and forehead.

- Remove cream with cleansing tissues or warm moist towel.
- Apply emollient cream according to the type of skin in the same manner as indicated above. Use lanolin or hormone cream for a dry skin and cold cream for an oily skin.
- For neck, face, shoulder and chest, apply emollient cream.
- Apply eye cream under the eyes gently with fingertips.
- Use muscle oil around the neck.
- For massaging face, apply massage cream giving manipulations with slightly cupped hands and fingers.
- Start massage under the lower lip with two fingers. Repeat process several times. Pinch gently along the jaw line, working outward towards ears.

How to get Beneficial Results from Massage?

- Early morning massage has a miraculous effect on the various organs.
- It is important to give massage in a comfortable environment. Choose a warm, peaceful place with dim lights and light music.
- Lie on a firm, padded surface while having massage, to relax the back and the stomach.
- Place a cushion under the knees to reduce the arch of the lower back and place a small cushion or folded towel under the head.
- A hard bed is ideal for a soothing massage, which can leave you relaxed and sleepy.
- Keep your back straight throughout the massage and use the weight of your body to give rhythm and depth.
- Never stay in one position when having massage.

- Keep your feet wide apart and bend the knees so that you can lean into the strokes.
- Wear loose-fitting washable clothes and be barefooted.
- Remove ornaments from your body before having massage, which can cause scratches.
- Support a sway back with a cushion under the waist.
- If you feel pain or an uncomfortable situation during massage, inform the masseur.
- Mould your hands to the contours of the face.
- Vary pressure from very light to very strong. The massage should be lighter over bony areas and firmer over the muscles.
- Do not apply heavy pressure when massaging.
- Concentrate on the massage. Avoid talking when massaging. Feel totally relaxed for a good massage.
- Do not worry if your initial movements seem clumsy. Practice will make you perfect.
- Deep pressure should not be used on swollen joints and nerves, which may increase inflammation.
- Avoid body massage in case of an infection or a contagious skin disease, high temperature, bruises or an acute inflammation, an inflammatory condition such as thrombosis or phlebitis, venereal diseases like diphtheria and gonorrhea—which cause formation of pus. A massage may spread the pus to entire system.
- During pregnancy, do not massage without consulting your doctor.

How to Massage the Face?

- For an effective massage, clean the facial skin.
- Start massage from the neck upward and end at the forehead or temples because all veins and tissues get blood circulation.
- Avoid pressing the delicate skin around the eyes.

- Massage for a minimum of 15-20 minutes as cream takes that much time to get absorbed.
- Always wipe off extra cream with a cotton swab.
- Wash hands with soap before starting massage.
- Remove all traces of stale or fresh make-up before massage otherwise the skin pores will get blocked.
- Remove blackheads before massage.
- Remove oiliness with cleansing milk or pH acid, if the skin is too oily. Use moisturizer before massage, if the skin is over dry. Use astringent lotion before massage, if the skin is damp and fleshy.
- The best time to massage a face is at night before sleep.

Rejuvenation Massage Therapies

- **Siddha, vaidya and ayurveda** are useful therapies in which special herbal oils are used by the massage, that trigger balance to the body. They affect the autonomic nervous system, the endocrine system, blood pressure, make body slim and trim, relieve stress, increase protein biosynthesis, elevate body enzymes synthesis, improve mental power, increase physical ability, fight free radicals, improve eyesight, beneficial to cardio-vascular and respiratory system. Shirodhara, nasaya, rasayanas, abhyanga (massage), svedana (steaming), sneha (application of pastes and masques), aromatherapy (massage with herbal oils), chromotherapy (treatment with color therapy), panchkarma (scientific system to detoxify and rejuvenate whole body), kriya karma (rejuvenation), purva karma, crystal and gem therapy, high frequency therapy (thermal heat produced due to rapid vibrations but without muscular contraction), shirobasti, akashi tarpan (treatment with medicated ghee or oil in eyes), juice therapy, sidha massage are some of naturopathic therapies beneficial for the body.

- **Micro therapy:** Also known as power massage therapy is used to treat ageing skin, laughing lines, frown lines etc. Being a very safe therapy, it is recommended for every age group. This therapy has the following benefits:
  1. Helps to improve blood circulation.
  2. Stimulates muscles and nerves.
  3. Regenerates cells and tissues.
  4. Used for face lifting.
  5. Promotes production of elastin fiber in the skin.
- **Derma brasion therapy:** This therapy helps to solve various skin problems and is basically done for leveling the surface of the skin. It is mostly given in case of uneven tone and cure blemishes, pigmentation, scars and acne marks. The damaged layer of the skin is replaced with the new layer of the skin. The therapy has the following benefits:
  1. Helps to level the crust.
  2. Helps in reducing facial scars.
  3. Helps in getting rid of ugly tans.
  4. Eradicates facial marks.
- **Ultrasonic massage therapy:** This therapy brings the glow back, improves circulation and is very effective to clear dull and sallow skin. The therapy is extremely beneficial in winter. It has the following benefits:
  1. Activates sebaceous glands.
  2. Improves dry skin.
  3. Improves blood circulation.
- **High frequency therapy:** This therapy, essentially a thermal heat treatment provides efficient and excellent results because of its rapid primary action without muscular contraction. This therapy helps curing various eye disorders and cure dark circles on the face.
- **Ozone therapy:** This therapy performed by using anti-allergic, antiseptic sterilized powder produces alkaline

rays, which are useful for the treatment of face and scalp. It is especially recommended for the treatment of acne, pimples, skin infections, excessive secretion of sebum etc. The therapy has the following benefits:

1. Controls hair dandruff.
2. Controls oil production and pus infection.
3. Treatment of thinning hair and itchy scalp.

- **Electric suction therapy:** This therapy is suitable for every age group and is capable to suck out infection, dirt, dust and germs from the epidermis (the outer layer of the skin). The electric suction therapy performed with the help of a compressor has the following benefits:

  1. Leaves an antiseptic effect on the skin.
  2. Improves blood circulation.
  3. Removes infection and reduces the growth of unfriendly bacteria.
  4. Helps in controlling sebum.
  5. Tightens skin pores.

Few Specialized Facial Massage Movements

- To soothe anxiety, headache and exhaustion, give your face a massage with a stroking movement. This improves poor circulation, relaxed muscles, removes lines and wrinkles, gives healthy and vibrant glow to the complexion. For a good massage, use sufficient lubrication, avoid dragging the skin, clean your hands before massage and file your nails to avoid scratching.
- Start massaging at the base of neck to chin. Continue massage under the jaw to the ears and work back under the chin.
- Stroke all over the face with your fingertips. Glide hands from chin to nostrils, the sides of the nose, below the eyes, under the cheekbones, up to the temples and back to the chin.

- Now stroke up to the bridge of the nose and continue across the forehead and to the temples, then glide down to the chin. Repeat the complete massage movements four to five times.
- Cup your hands over the face with palms on the forehead and fingers over the mouth. Press down and hold for few seconds, then release the pressure and remove your hands. Repeat movements four to five times. You will feel fresh.
- Perform neck massage with both hands stroking from the shoulder to the ear. Stimulate the jaw line by patting and strapping under the chin and under the jaw line using middle fingers Repeat movements four to five times.
- For massaging the cheeks, make upward, circular, smooth movements all over the face with loose fingertips of both hands and crossed thumbs. Stroke your fingertips on the upper lip, under the cheekbones, around and under the lower tip of ears and the jaws. This movement releases tension in the facial muscles.
- To massage forehead, apply pressure with the first two fingers of each hand in circles. These soothing movements reduce tension and headache. Upward circular movements energize, while downward circular movements give relaxation and relieve tension.
- To remove wrinkles under the eyes, start massage gently at the bridge of the nose, stroking lightly along the eyebrows with fingertips and glide towards temples, then back to under the eyes and nose. Do not forget to squeeze the eyebrows between your thumbs and forefingers during under eye massage.
- To finish facial massage, cup your hands over the forehead. Hold for few seconds, then press down gently, release pressure gradually and slowly remove the hands from the forehead. This will ease tension from the body.

Essential Oil Facial Massage

Essential oil is beneficial for massaging the face, neck and décolleté area for the below mentioned reasons. Facial massage should be no longer than 15-20 minutes. The massage movements should be light but positive:

- It stimulates the blood supply, which increases the oxygen level and improves the skin tone.
- It increases the circulatory flow and the warmth in the dermis of skin due to massage movements allows greater absorption of the essential oils.
- It relaxes facial muscle tension and softens the facial expression under stress condition.
- It stimulates the lymphatic flow in the area, which help speed up the elimination of cellular waste matter, toxins and other impurities.
- It helps dispel tiredness.

Analysis of the Skin

Carry out analysis of the skin to help selection of the correct essential oil as well as techniques of right massage movements:

• **Pale skin**	Indicate poor blood circulation or a medical condition such as anemia or low blood pressure.
• **Discoloured skin**	Indicate toxicity or previous bruising.
• **Yellow skin**	Indicate kidney or liver problems.
• **Bluish tinge**	Indicate poor blood circulation.
• **Cold hands/ feet**	Indicate poor blood circulation.
• **Varicose veins**	Indicate colon problems, back problems, lack of exercise, stagnant energy and fluid flow.
• **Spongy tissue**	Indicate water retention or poor nutrition.

• **Muscles tension**	Indicate tension caused by injury, stress or holding the body in a fixed position.
• **Knotted tissue**	May indicate scar tissue or congestion.
• **Hard skin**	Indicate crystallization.
• **Congested skin**	Indicate crystallization.
• **Thick toe nails**	Indicate fungal, rheumatic condition.

Procedure for Facial Massage

This massage conducted on facial reflex points carried on both sides of the face, neck and shoulder. The following steps are advised:

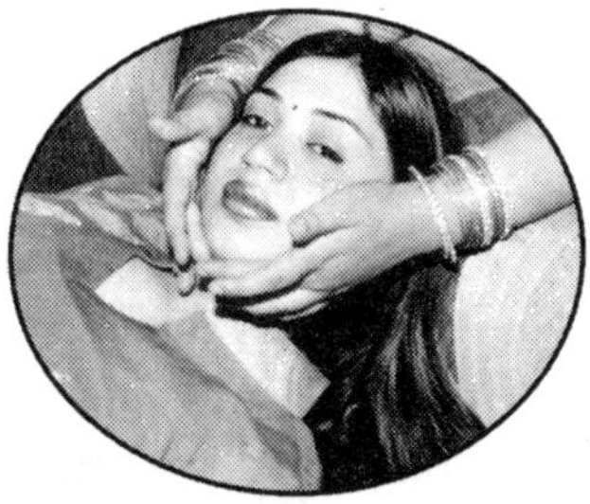

- Warm your hands by rubbing them together so that warm energy start flowing through them.
- Pour little massage oil on the palm and rub both hands.
- Start massaging the face in sections from chin towards the forehead. Gently place the hands on the muscle and move towards the occipital bone in a continuous flowing movement.

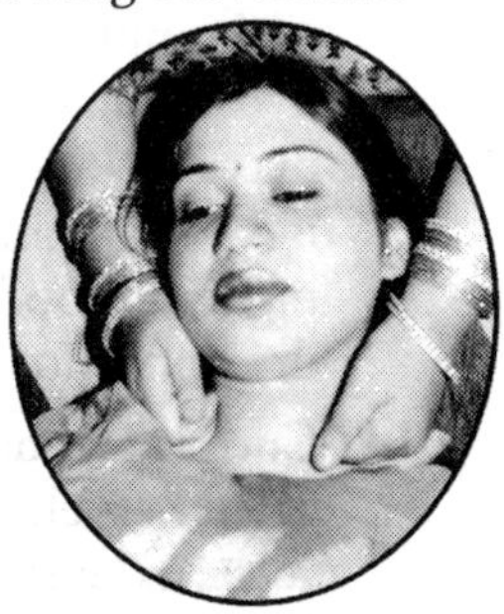

- Start massage with the right hand, followed by the left. Pour a little massage oil into your hand. Use light effleurage movements upwards over the face traveling movements with the middle finger.
- Massage face with gentle pressure and small circular, stationary movements. Take cheek muscles between your thumb and index fingers, and gently squeeze,

moving underneath the cheekbone. Rest for five seconds with both hands on the face.

- Apply smooth upward movements along the sides of the face, starting at the chin and ending at the temples. Now harmonize energy by holding the face in the hands for few seconds.
- Apply face pack matching the texture of your skin. Leave it on for ten minutes, then remove the pack and apply moisturizer.
- Relax for few minutes and have a glass of water.

Functioning of Massage Oils

Oils play an important role and cover 'top to toe' beauty of body. There are three varieties of oils:

- Basic or original oils, which are pure vegetable extracts.
- Processed or commercial oils prepared with analytical combinations of various necessary ingredients.
- Synthetic oils, which have different uses in their various ranges.

Almond, coconut, sesame, castor and olive oil are commonly used varieties of oils available in India to enhance beauty of skin and scalp. The following are cosmetic and pharmaceutical properties of these oils:

- **Almond (badam) oil:** These are of two types: sweet and bitter. Bitter almond contains traces of hydrodynamic acid and is not recommended for facial massage. Sweet almond oil is used for face massage to improve complexion, prevent wrinkles, remove eye make-up, body massage, healing chapped lips and for dry and brittle hair.
- **Coconut (nariyal) oil:** This oil extracted from the dried kernel, contains 60-70% oil. The oil has benefits such as cure skin diseases, leprosy cure, used for thickness and growth of hair.
- **Sesame (til) oil:** Sesame seeds are of three types—white, red and black. The white seeds possess

maximum oil. The oil extracted from black seeds has medicinal properties and contains 50-60% oil. It softens rough skin, used in formulations for massage in paralytic conditions, clears facial skin, used for body massage and growth of hair.

- **Olive (jaitun) oil:** A good conditioner and helps growth and thickness of hair.

Facial Reflex Points

Pressing reflex points on the face increase energy flow and leads to revitalization. The movements are carried out at the end of a facial. Press each point in sequence for a few seconds in a gentle press-and-lift movement on both side of the face at the same time. Pressing these points helps to improve circulation and energy flow in the face and also tones the skin. Hold each point for five seconds.

- **If the face looks tired or is sagging,** rub at the centre of lower cheekbone on both sides of the face.
- **In case of puffy eyes,** rub on either side of the nose.
- **If the face looks tired or is sagging,** rub at the outer corners of the eyes on both sides.
- **In case of droopy cheeks and jowls,** rub the hollow just below the ears on both sides of the face.
- **In case of eye bags and loose cheek muscles,** rub border line between the eye socket and cheekbone on both sides of the face.
- **To tone up muscles of entire body and energize them,** rub at the centre of the palms of both hands.

Important Movements of Facial Reflex Points

- **Press points on the bridge of nose, between the eyes and at the bottom of the forehead:** Use both the thumbs one following the other.
- **Press point above the eyebrow, at the centre of the face, along the line of eyebrows and outwards until complete forehead has been covered:** Start at the

centre and smooth towards the temples with the finger of both hands.

- **Press under the inner eyebrows, press inline outwards up to the outer corner of the eyes:** Press adjacent to the outer corner of the eyes.
- **Press at either side of the nose and upper lip:** Work outwards towards the ear under the cheekbone.
- **Press between the nose and upper lip:** Press outwards in a continuous line.
- **Press under the lower lip:** Press outwards in a continuous line with two fingers.
- **Pinch pressure point gently along the jaw line:** Work outwards.
- **Press along the entire hairline:** Work towards the ears.

Precautions when having Facial Massage

The following precautions should be taken for a facial massage:

- Hands should not be removed from the face once the manipulations have started.
- Massage movements are usually directed towards the origin of a muscle in order to avoid damage to muscular tissue.
- Make sure that the skin is clean before starting massage, because massage is effective if the skin is clean.
- The massage should start from the neck upwards and end at the forehead or temples, because all veins and tissues get blood circulation by this process.
- Massage for 15 to 20 minutes as the massage cream takes that much time to get absorbed.
- Wash hands with the soap before starting massaging.
- Avoid pressing delicate skin around the eyes.
- Remove make up completely before massaging, otherwise the skin pores get blocked by the make up particles.

- If there are blackheads on the skin, remove before massage.
- If the skin is excessive oily, apply cleansing milk or lemon juice or pH acid before massage.
- If the skin is over-dry, use moisturizer before the massage.
- If the skin is damp, use astringent lotion before massage.
- As far as possible, massage before going to bed at night.
- If the facial skin is fleshy, use slimming cream.

Some of the prominent movements for facial massage are given below:

- **Linear movement:** Apply with fingers rotating with an upward pressure stroke usually on forehead and temples.
- **Circular movement:** Start at the eyebrow line and move towards the hairline.
- **Criss-cross movement:** Start at the side of forehead and work back.
- **Stroking movement:** Slide fingers over brows on forehead and move towards temples with slight pressure.
- **Brow and eye movement:** Place middle fingers at inner corners of the eyes and index fingers over brows. Slide towards outer corners of eyes under eyes, and back to inner corners of eyes
- **Nose and upper cheek movement:** Slide fingers down the nose applying rotary movement across the cheeks and temples rotating gently.
- **Mouth and nose movement:** Apply circular movement from corners of the mouth towards the upside of nose and brows and down to the mouth.
- **Lip and chin movement:** Draw fingers from centre of upper lip towards lower lip and chin.

- **Optional movement:** Draw right hand finger under lower lip, centre of upper lip and round the mouth.
- **Lifting movement of cheeks:** Proceed from the mouth to ear and nose to ear on cheeks.
- **Rotational movement:** Massage from chin to earlobes, moth to middle of ears and nose to top of ears on the cheeks.
- **Light tapping movement:** Work from chin to earlobe, mouth to ear, nose to top of ear and across the forehead on both sides of the face.
- **Stroking movement:** Apply light upward strokes over the neck, applying downward strokes in the front and pressure on the sides and the back of neck.
- **Circular movement:** Start at the back of ears applying circular movement over shoulders and across the chest.
- **Pinching movement:** The skin to be massaged is held between the thumb and fingers as in pincers. It is very useful in case of eradicating jaw wrinkles and for double skin.
- **Fast massage movement:** Massaging with the front halves of both the palms in upward, circular motion. It helps in removing wrinkles.
- **Pressure movement:** Massage is applied with fleshy fingertips. It is useful for removing pouches under the eyes.

Facial Exercises

The object of doing facial exercise is to improve and strengthen the muscles and to increase blood circulation. Practice each exercise for six to ten times. There are six types of facial exercises:

- Open your mouth wide as if you are going to scream. Open eyes wide, stare and revert to the original position.

- Press your forehead near the hairline with your fingers and massage it with backward motion. This exercise helps to remove the creases on the forehead.
- Open your mouth wide and slide head back. Now open and close your mouth as in munching.
- Turn your lips inwards. Fill your mouth with air and try bringing a smile on one half of your face. Repeat the same exercise on the other half of the face. This exercise will smoothen your cheeks.
- Press your teeth and spread your lips, keeping your face straight. Hold for few seconds and revert to normal pose.
- Twist lips and puff up your cheeks. Keep three fingers on each side of the face and press slowly without letting the air out. Remain in this position till you can. This is very effective exercise for cheeks and mouth.
- Clench teeth hard and turn your lips inside. Stretch the corners of your mouth as much as possible so that it seems you are grimacing. Hold for few seconds and relax for a while. Push the lower jaw as far forward as you can and relax. This facial exercise is beneficial for flabby jaw line.
- Sit straight facing the mirror. Look at the ceiling stretching your neck. Now turn your head and look over your left shoulder. Remain in this position for some time and return to initial position. Now look over your right shoulder and return to normal position. Relax for some time and repeat exercise as many times as you can. This exercise relieves a double chin.

5

Body Massage to Control Ageing

Massage to Fight Ageing

Massage is one of the easiest ways for attaining and maintaining health, youth, vigour and beauty. Aches, pains, insomnia (lack of sleep), tension and stress can be alleviated with a simple instrument—hands. Many experts advise couples to touch each other more often as this can prevent physical and mental illness in a human body. Massage improves circulation, relaxes muscles, aids digestion by stimulating the lymphatic system, eliminates the waste products and toxins in the body, provides energy and refreshes the body. Early morning massage has a miraculous effect on the various organs.

How to Get Beneficial Effects from Massage?

- To get good results, it is important that the massage should be given in a comfortable environment. Select a warm, calm place with dim lights.
- Always lie on a firm, padded surface to relax the back and the stomach. Always place a cushion under the knees to reduce the arch of the lower back. Place a small cushion or folded towel under the head to raise it about one to three inches.
- In case of giving a soothing massage, use a bed which can leave you relaxed and sleepy.

- Keep your back straight throughout the massage and use the weight of the body to give rhythm and depth to the massage.
- Keep your feet wide apart during massage and bend the knees so that you can lean into the strokes. In case you are working on the floor, kneel with your knees apart.
- Never stay in one position for a long while massaging.
- Wear loose fitting, washable clothes during massage. Avoid wearing shoes; wear flat shoes or be bare-footed.
- Remove all gold/silver/diamond ornaments from the body before giving the massage, as they may cause scratches on the skin while giving massage.
- When massaging the back, put a small cushion or rolled towel under the ankles.
- For a relaxing massage, put a cushion under the waist and put another cushion under the shoulder.
- Remember, a firm, brisk massage is invigorating whereas slow, steady massage strokes lead to sleep. Do not repeat the same massage twice.

Massage Techniques

- A rhythmic massage sends waves of relaxation throughout the body.
- If you feel pain or uncomfortable during massage, inform the masseur.
- Mould your hands to the contours of the body.
- Vary pressure from very light to very strong.
- Massage lightly over the bony areas and firmly over the muscles.
- Do not apply heavy pressure when massaging.
- Avoid talking while massaging. Concentrate only on massage.
- Be totally relaxed when giving a massage.

- Do not worry if your initial massage movements seem clumsy. Practice makes one perfect.

Do not massage if you are suffering from:

- An infection, a contagious disease of the skin.
- High temperature.
- A skin infection, bruises or acute inflammation (such as thrombosis or phlebitis).
- Serious inflammatory cases of the joints and in tubercular joints.
- In case of infectious diseases like diphtheria and gonorrhea, which cause formation of pus. Massage may spread the pus to the entire system.

Basic Body Massage Movements

Kneading and percussion strokes cause muscles to contract and become stronger. Deep circular kneading and vibration strokes loosen the muscles. Kneading under and round the muscles breaks adhesions. Massage benefits many nerve problems. In case of acute inflammation of the nerves, massage should be done carefully by light and gentle strokes. Do not apply deep pressure on swollen nerves; it can increase inflammation. Just a gentle beating of the nerve is enough. Nerve compression is recommended for soothing nerves.

Spinal nerve compression is extremely beneficial in case of insomnia (loss of sleep). It is done with the palms; the vibration of the fingers stimulates spinal nerves. Abdominal massage is beneficial in constipation and stimulates peristalsis of the small intestines, tones up muscles of the abdominal walls. Abdominal massage should not be done in case of inflammation of the uterus, bladder, ovaries and fallopian tubes, when suffering from stone in kidney or gall bladder, ulcer of the stomach and intestines, in case of pregnancy and after taking a heavy meal.

To do abdominal massage, the bladder should be emptied before a massage. The patient is made to lie on the back with knees drawn up to enable the abdominal wall to relax.

Chest massage is helpful in many ways. It strengthens the chest muscles, increases circulation and tones up the nerves system of the chest, heart and lungs. It is especially recommended in case of weak lungs, palpitation and organic heart disorders. Chest massage helps to develop bust and mammary glands. Massage is a method of manipulating the soft tissue of the body. There are five classical massage movements as below:

Massage for Expected Mothers

Careful, smooth and gentle massage movements should be applied, which benefit a woman during pregnancy. Do not forget to consult a doctor before applying massage to an expectant woman. Massage helps alleviate many complications such a tension, backache, insomnia (sleeplessness) and fatty deposits on the body. A pregnant woman should avoid a deep pressure and percussion movements. A careful massage before conception helps to increase the fertility, and three months before the delivery makes labour painless.

You may use all types of movement recommended for abdomen, back, shoulder, leg and feet massage in gentle and very light movements. Use cushion under the shoulder, lower back and knees to reduce curves and discomfort while massaging. Massage done by the trained masseuse makes childbirth easier. Lower back and shoulders are the areas, which relieve tension when massaging. For a back massage, a pregnant should lie on her side. Or sit on a chair, facing towards the back of chair. The following massage movements are beneficial for a pregnant:

1. Apply gentle stroking firstly with one hand, then with both hands one following other clockwise on the abdomen.
2. Stroke softly on the side of the waist upwards with one hand after the other till both hands reach the navel. Now gently glide the hands towards the abdomen downward, and then to the sides to complete the stroke.
3. Cup your hands over the navel for few seconds till you feel the heat. Slowly remove hands.

4. Leg massage, too, is very beneficial for pregnant women. It soothes, relaxes and relieves swelling and pain in legs, cures varicose veins and leg cramps usually faced by expectant mothers.
5. The best remedy is to sleep with the legs slightly raised above the level of head, which relieves swelling in the legs.
6. Massage purifies and corrects drainage system of the body, melts fat deposits, calms the nerves, drains waste products and toxins and cures many skin disorders like eczema, acne, dermatitis etc. related with pregnancy.
7. Light stroking movements may be applied on the mid back just above the waist, at the base of spine and between the shoulder blades on the back of an expecting mother.
8. Press firmly applying circular pressure with your thumbs on the hips and buttocks to relieve lower back pain and melt fat deposits on the hips and thighs.
9. Foot massage pressing few shiatsu points can relieve pain during labour and help speedy delivery. Stroke the sole of the feet firmly with the heel of your hand. Apply deep pressure with thumbs in the center of the sole to the heel of the feet, which reduce labour pains.

Massage after the Childbirth

A deep massage to abdomen for 40 days after the delivery of baby energizes the mother, cures body aches and brings uterus back to its original position. The following abdominal massage movements should be applied:

1. Stroke abdomen in all directions. Knead firmly on hips and gently across the abdomen.
2. Stroke clockwise in large circles on the abdomen applying gentle pressure.

3. Stroke slowly up the abdomen starting at the pubic bone and pressing with heels of hands.
4. Stroke slowly on the lower abdomen starting from the pubic bone to the navel.
5. Finally cup your hands over the navel and hold for few seconds until you feel heat accumulating beneath the hands. Now lift hands slowly.

Neck and Chin Massage

Neck massage is essential as the nerves of this region have to support the weight of head, which weighs between five to seven kilograms. The following movements stimulate the circulation of neck muscles and prevent development of double chin. Neck massage includes the following massage movements:

1. Stroke from the collarbone to chin using back of your hands to massage one side, one hand following the other. Now repeat this movement to the other side.
2. Pinch along your jaw line with thumbs and knuckles of your fingers, starting from chin to the ears without stretching.
3. Slap gently under the chin with your hands alternately. This will stimulate the muscles under the chin.
4. Now stroke from the corners of your mouth towards the ears with one hand on each cheek.
5. Press the temples under your fingers, clenching your teeth to stimulate the jaw muscles.

Shoulder Massage

The shoulder muscles usually remain tense and a massage relaxes them. The following massage movements should be carried:

- Start from the top of the shoulder up towards the sides of the neck. Mould your hands round the shoulders, gliding them with smooth and even pressure. Then slide down and repeat the movement four to five times.

- Knead the muscles gently working from shoulders.

Back Massage

Back massage leaves a relaxing effect, lowers stress level, cures back or spinal or body pain, induces a blissful state, relieves tense and knotted muscles. Back massage is beneficial for the entire nervous system. To do a back massage, the following steps are suggested:

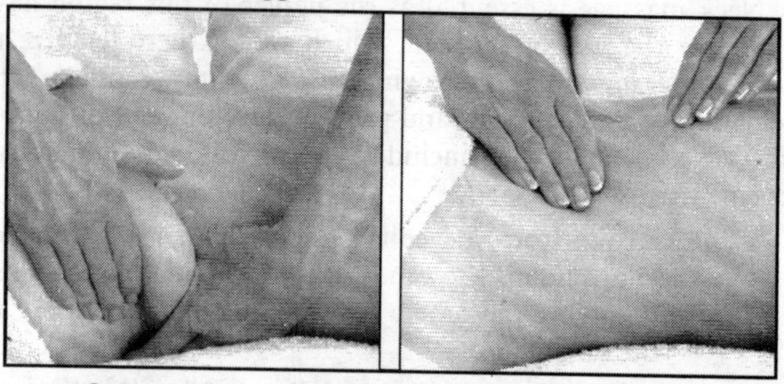

- Start with a stroking movement on the lower back with thumbs on either side of the spine and fingers pointing towards the head with relaxed hands. Stroke firmly up the back, then pull down on the muscles at the base of the neck, stroke across the shoulders on the upper arms on the curves of shoulders. Now glide hands tightly downwards on both sides of the back till the hands reach the waist. Repeat 10 to 12 times.

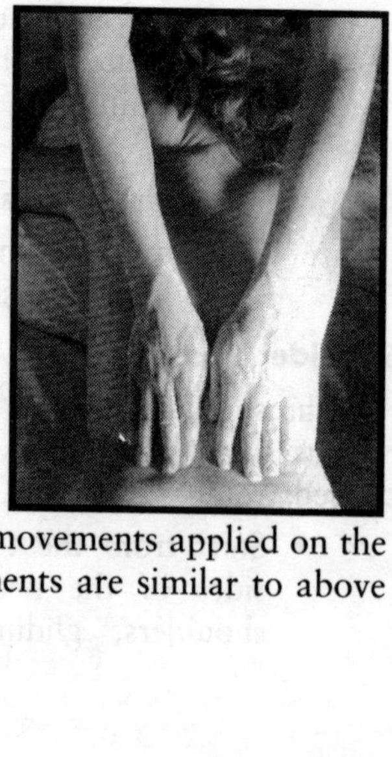

- Fan stroking or alternate stroking, too, are beneficial movements applied on the back massage. These movements are similar to above stroking movement to improve circulation, warm and soothe the skin.

- Kneading massage movement includes massage with both hands facing each other, squeezing the flesh with both hands. Start at the hips and work up the sides of the body on one side followed by the other. Continue kneading movements at the back of the neck, shoulders and upper arms to relieve tensed skin tissues.
- Side stroking is a movement to stroke up at the side of the back with loose, released hand pulling in towards the spine with one hand following the other in a smooth, flowing rhythm.
- To perform circle stroking, place both hands on one side of the back. Slide one hand downwards on the same side in a curve and the other hand up to the spine. Continue stroking in circles clockwise. Then shift the movement on the other side in anticlockwise direction.
- While doing pressure stroking, relax muscles on either side of the spine with firm pressure exerted by the pads of the thumbs. Start at the lower back, press firmly, release and repeat at the other place in upward direction till the hands reach the shoulder and base of the neck. It is very beneficial for the shoulder muscles. Brisk movements bring blood to the nerves, which ease pain and tiredness.
- Circle thumb stroking is a movement similar to circle stroking, but the stroke is applied with thumbs instead of palms.

Buttocks Massage

Tension usually exists at the lower back and the buttocks. Bottom is the most neglected area of the body. Buttock muscles can get rid of tension with powerful massage movements as below:

- Work flowing and rhythmic strokes in circles clockwise on right buttock and anticlockwise on the left buttock, gliding downwards.

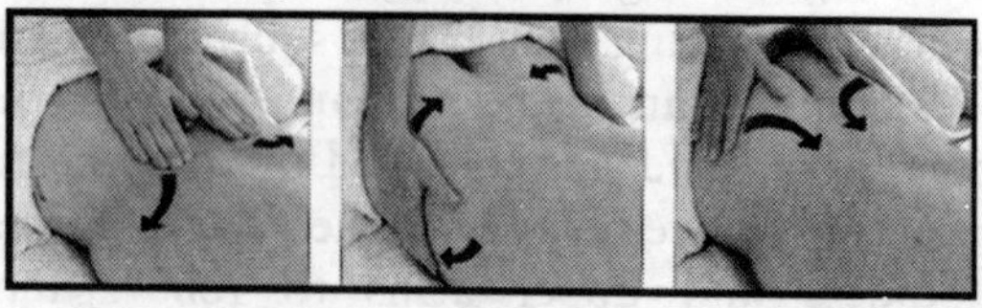

- Place hands on the buttocks and stroke smoothly up towards sideways with relaxed hands, then twisting inwards from the sides of the waist. Now push the hands up, kneading fleshy buttocks in hands. Repeat movements several times.
- Apply circular pressure with thumbs of both hands at the bony base of the spine.

Spine Massage

The spine is built of small bones called vertebrae, which are stacked up in a column having spongy pads (known as discs) between the bones. The spinal cord is a bunch of nerve fibers running down a channel through the spine. The vertebrae mounted on the solid base is attached to the pelvis. To do spine massage, the following steps are recommended:

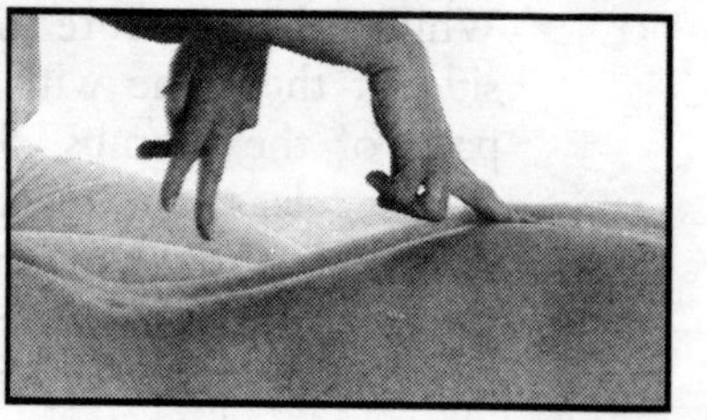

- Start massaging at the neck with index and middle fingers on either side of the spine. Make firm strokes downwards on the back with both hands one after the other.
- Now place right hand at the base of spine, resting middle of the palm on the bone of the spinal cord and press the spine with the middle finger. Do not press hard on the vertebrae.
- Apply stretching movement. Cross arms and place one hand on the sacrum and the other hand on the centre

of the spinal cord with hands facing away from each other.

- Now apply a diagonal stretch to the back, placing one hand on the shoulder and other on the hip. After massaging for some time, repeat movement on the other shoulder.

Thigh Massage

The following massage movements are beneficial for thighs:

- **Stroking:** Stroke up the back of thighs firmly towards hips with one hand and glide back down to the knees. Do it simultaneously with other hand. This helps to improve the shape of the thighs and is very soothing.

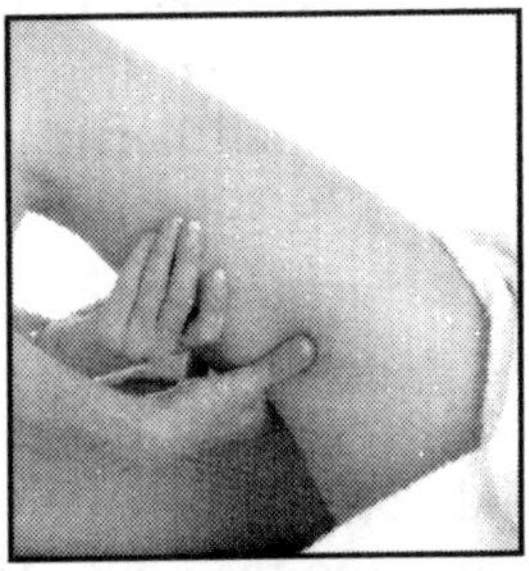

- **Criss-crossing the thighs:** Start movement behind the thigh, placing hands on the top of the thigh and fingers curling on the sides. Squeeze the muscles by gliding your hands in all directions.
- **Thumb circling:** Stroke gently, knees cupped in the fingers of both hands. Now glide each thumb in the opposite direction to do a complete circle round the knees.
- **Rotary pressure stroking:** Gently stroke the fingers around the knee applying pressure with your thumbs. Stroke up massaging towards the thigh and make gentle, rotary movements behind the knee. Massage thighs with stroking, kneading, criss-crossing and pummeling movements.
- **Rolling:** This movement improves skin texture and release tension. Place hands on outer thighs touching fingers and thumb together. Now roll the flesh by pinching the skin smoothly between the thumb and fingers.

- **Passive movements:** Flex the knee and hip gently after the massage has been finished to relax the leg muscles. Hold ankle and knee, kneel over the hips, bend the knee lifting the leg up and rotate the hip joint. Repeat three to four times in each direction. Do not apply heavy force on knee joint.
- **For getting extra relaxing effect:** Relax for a moment straightening the leg, lower it smoothly supporting the knee and ankle. Apply knuckling movement by curling your hands into loose fists with middle section of fingers against the skin. Then grabble and release small portions of the flesh quickly with thumbs and forefingers on the thighs.

Foot Massage

Foot massage not only relaxes thousands of nerve endings existing in the sole, but also refreshes and stimulates the whole body. The feet contain almost 25% of all the bones and muscles in the body. These bones and muscles help the foot to support the weight of the body and provide leverage when walking. These are basically of three types as below:

- Main.
- High arch, which runs along the inside edge of the foot.
- Lower arch, which run along the outside edge across the base of the toes.

Fine quality excessive oil is required to massage feet, which makes the fingers slide over the skin. The following strokes are applied to enjoy a foot massage:

- **Stroking movement:** Start massage by stroking the foot firmly between the hands from toes towards the ankles and back to toes to warm up the feet. Repeat for four to five times.
- **Thumb stroking:** Stroke up the foot with your thumbs on the top and base of the toe supporting the foot with fingers. Glide thumbs to massage up to the ankle.

- **Toe massage:** Rotate the hands wiggling the toes. Massage each toe individually, squeezing and rolling the toe. Massage thoroughly on the base of the toe.
- Finally, support the foot between both hands and stroke between the tendons—one thumb following the other.

For giving a brisk foot massage, the following specialized movements are necessary:

- **Pressure:** Press firmly on the sole holding the foot with fingers on top and thumbs underneath the foot for six to eight seconds. Apply pressure on the ball of the foot.
- **Arch stroking:** Stimulate and soothe the foot by stroking resting one hand on the top of the foot and stroking the ball of the foot with the other hand.
- **Kneading:** Keep one hand on the top of the foot and stroking firmly all over the sole with the middle section of the finger of other hand.
- **Applying rotary pressure:** Stroke the whole foot. Then apply circular upward pressures all round the ankles with one hand on each side of the feet.
- **Hacking movements:** Hold the foot firmly with one hand and hack the sole with the side of other hand keeping it flexible. Now use both hands to hack the sole as well as top of the feet with faster movement.
- **Passive movements:** Support the ankle of the feet with one hand, loosen the muscles of the whole feet and ankle with gentle passive movements and slowly flex the feet up and down four to five times in each direction. Repeat movements on the other feet.
- To end the foot massage, stroke the whole foot after vigorous movement with both hands up towards the ankles. This sequence leaves the foot feeling soothed. Finally glide your hands slowly towards the toes. Repeat massage movements three to four times.

Leg Massage

Legs are built to carry the weight of the body. Legs are sturdy with strong muscles and bones. The knee joint is strengthened by the knee cap—a circular bone, which helps the knee to carry body weight. Deep, firm massage on the muscles of the leg helps to dispel fatigue. Leg massage bring blood and nutrients to the leg muscles and relieve tightness, cramps and prevent varicose veins. Do not forget to press lightly over the bony areas and knees. In case one is suffering from the varicose veins, massage very gently, avoiding heavy movements such as kneading and pummeling. Do not press over the affected vein. Gently stroke up the legs in the direction of the lymph nodes, which usually exist at the back of knees and in the groin. Massaging legs and feet helps reduce puffiness or swelling in legs, cure aggravated backache or pain. Leg massage lying on the back is very beneficial. The following massage movements should be applied on the legs:

- **Stroking the legs:** Cup the hands over the ankles and stroke up on all sides of the bone. Press sides of the legs towards the thighs and lower legs with the heels of hands.
- **Kneading the calf:** Support the ankles with one hand and knead the calf muscles with the other hand. Press the flesh between palms and fingers and squeeze the muscles till the hands glide up to the knees. Now glide back towards the ankles releasing the pressure. Repeat massage movements several times.
- **Stroking up the calf:** Supporting the ankles, bend knees to rest the feet flat on the floor. Stroke firmly and smoothly up the calf and pull muscles upward and to the sides gliding hands up and down.
- **Criss-crossing the calf:** This massage movement releases tension in the calf muscles and benefits those who stand for a long time. Avoid this movement if you are suffering from varicose veins. Work from the ankles to the knees and back. Place your hands round the calf and leg. The thumb should be at the front and

fingers on the sides. Do not pinch the flesh when massaging.

The movement for massaging back of legs is similar to those used for massaging the front of legs as following:

- Stroke the leg from ankles to thighs. Press gently over the knee.
- Knead the calf muscle using both hands.
- Stroke up the calf with thumbs, pressing firmly.
- Stress gently on the back of knee, using fingers.
- Stroke up the thigh from the knee, pummeling the outer thigh.
- Lift the feet up, supporting with the other hand.
- Stroke the whole leg, stimulating by hacking the side of the feet with the edge of the hand.
- Lower the leg and finish massage movements by stroking leg gently.

Hand Massage

Hands are one of the most sensitive parts of the body, which contain large number of nerve endings linked to the brain to register sensation of the whole body. To ease stiff and tired muscles of the hand, a regular hand massage is beneficial. If hands are neglected, skin of the hands becomes aged and wrinkled. Massaging the hands with cream or oil and moisturizing them stimulates the blood supply and keeps them soft and supple. Hand massage can be given anywhere without inconvenience of getting undressed. The following are common movements of a hand massage:

- Stroking the palm with the heel of the other hand.
- Thumb stroking towards the wrist.
- Stretching the fingers.

The following movements are suggested for a hand massage:

- Stroke in furrows between the tendons with your thumb towards the wrist, one thumb following the other.

- Move your fist all over the palm, making circular movements with knuckle of your fingers.
- Continue to stretch the palm of the hand after you interlock your fingers in it, making circular pressure massage with the thumb to ease tension from the hands.
- Give wrist massage holding the hand in the fingers. Stroke towards the arm and out to the sides with thumbs.
- To give final touches to hand massage, stroke the whole hand between the palms of your hands and press firmly for a few seconds. Release pressure and slide your hands slowly off the fingers leaving the hands fully relaxed.

Finger Massage

Fingers though small and bony, too, need a massage. Hold palm down with one hand and use the other hand to work on each finger, stroking from the tip to the knuckle, followed by squeezing the entire finger. Apply circular pressure round each joint of the finger with thumb. Do not jerk the fingers, stretch it gently to ease the joints. Complete the massage routine applying circular pressure deeply on the thumb and the muscular area at the base of the thumb.

Arm Massage

The bones of arms and hands are much delicate than those of the legs and feet. Usually, arms are neglected altogether. Remember, tension and tiredness in the arms leads to headache, neck pain and arching shoulders. A regular arm massage alleviates many body disorders. The techniques of arm massage are similar to those used in leg massage. The following massage movements are suggested for an arm massage:

- Start with stroking movements firmly across the wrist up the arms with slightly cupped hands to exert deep pressure on the muscles and light pressure over the bones. When you reach the shoulder joint, open your hands and glide them lightly downward till you reach the back of the wrist. Repeat massage movements six to eight times.

- Now support the forearm with one hand and stroke up the arm with the other till the hand reaches the shoulder. Then glide hand downward. Repeat massage movement six to eight times.
- Fan stroking is conducted on inside the wrist with thumbs—one gliding up and the other down covering the entire forearm. Clasp your hands round the wrist to drain out the waist product from the veins sliding out one hand down to the elbow, pressing with thumb. Then glide back to the wrist. Make stroke firmly with your thumbs on inside of the wrist and cover the entire forearm.

Forearm, Elbow and Upper Arm Massage

The pumping movement of kneading ensures the arm is totally relaxed. To do this massage, rest hands on your thighs, knead the forearm gently with one hand working from wrist to the elbow and back. Repeat massage movement a couple of times. Know knead the same area with both hands.

To do elbow massage, support the arm with one hand and stroke the elbow with the other hand smoothly in circle with the tips of your fingers. Apply circular pressure all over the elbow with plenty of oil, since elbows are often neglected parts of the body. Finish massage by stroking movements to soothe the skin.

For upper arm massage, the following movements are done:

- **Stroke from elbow upwards to the shoulder.** Press shoulders gently and stroke with other hand. Massage with the first hand downward and repeat.
- **Support the arm with one hand.** Knead the upper arm on both sides with the other hand. When the arm is heavy (bulky), you may have to knead with the both hands, wringing and squeezing the flesh without hurting or pinching.

- **Feather stroking:** Stroke arm with both hands. Clasp the wrist and stretch arms gently. Finish by massaging your hands slowly off the fingers.
- **Passive movement:** Hold wrist with one hand and lift the arm up over the head, stretching it as far as possible comfortably. Slide your one hand down to the hip to give a long stretch. Shake the arm gently up and down and finish with a gentle pull. Make a large circle with the upper arm to rotate the shoulder joint, which makes the arm relaxed.

6

Antioxidants: Nutrients to Fight Ageing

The Theories of Ageing

There are many theories why we age and why only few of us reach out full calendar potential. Most of these theories fall into two main categories as below:

- **Damage theory:** Based on the premise that our life essence gets worn out, rusted and falls apart like an old vehicle or outdated appliance.
- **The pre-programmed theory:** Which indicates that we are stuck with a future and cannot control our lifetime, which has been set.

Life Expectancy Chart

The life span of a human being has been determined as 120 years, but life expectancy has been observed as 75 years. The chart below tells the average life expectancy in either the men's or women's according to National Centre of Health Statistics.

Age range years	Average remaining years of life for a male	Average remaining years of life for a female
0-1	71.8	78.6
1-5	71.6	78.3
5-10	67.8	74.4
10-15	62.8	69.5

Contd...

Age range years	Average remaining years of life for a male	Average remaining years of life for a female
15-20	57.9	64.6
20-25	53.3	59.7
25-30	48.7	54.9
30-35	44.1	50.1
35-40	39.6	45.3
40-45	35.1	40.5
45-50	30.7	35.8
50-55	26.4	31.3
55-60	22.3	26.9
60-65	18.6	22.7
65-70	15.2	18.8
70-75	12.1	15.2
75-80	9.4	11.9
80-85	7.1	9.0
85 +	5.3	6.6

Free Radicals and Metabolism

It is estimated that our bodies suffer 10,000 free radicals that hit our body everyday. It is similar to a piece of apple cut up and left for sometime, it becomes brownish or like a piece of un-painted iron bar, which gets rusted when exposed to oxygen.

Metabolism is a series of chemical reactions, which utilizes the nutrients for growth, repair or energy production within the body. The metabolism is the rate at which the body uses energy for the process of metabolism. The energy is measured in kilocalories (kcal) or kilojoules. One calorie is the amount of energy required to raise the temperature of 1 kg of water by 1 degree C. The joule is the metric unit of measurement for heat and energy (1 kcal : 4.2 kj). The graph below shows energy value of the nutrients.

Nutrients	Energy value
Carbohydrates	3.75 kcal (16 kj)
Protein	4.00 kcal (17 kj)
Fat	9.00 kcal (37 kj)

Energy Requirement

The amount of food, which a person requires in a day depend on the energy used during the day. This varies according to age, sex, body structure, occupation, physical activities and other conditions e.g. pregnancy or feeding a baby. In fact, ideally the food eaten each day should supply no more and no less than the amount of energy used in that day. The average energy requirement for an adult woman is approximately 1940 kcal and for a male 2550 kcal. Occupations are classified as follows according to how active they are:

- **Sedentary:** Office workers, clerical tasks, teachers and shopkeepers.
- **Moderate active:** Hairdressers, beauticians and a postman.
- **Very active:** Construction labourer, athletes, and hockey/football players.

What is metabolic rate?: A chemical process in which the cells are nourished and supplied with energy to carry on many activities in human body. In a healthy body, the metabolic rate is kept under control by a secretion from the thyroid gland. This can be called 'first you eat, then you die theory'. Every human being or animal uses up the same amount of chemical energy or calories in their life times. A mouse will burn the same number of calories per kilogram in a lifetime of one year as an elephant burns in 20 years.

There are two phases of metabolism:

- **Catabolism:** A destructive process, which breaks down larger substances or molecules into smaller ones. This process releases energy that can be stored by special molecules to be used for muscle contraction, secretion and heat production.
- **Anabolism:** A constructive process which build up larger molecules from smaller ones. During this process, the body stores water, food and oxygen to the time when these substances are needed for cell growth and repair.

Both anabolism and catabolism are carried out simultaneously in the cells so that their activities are closely regulated and balanced with building up and energy consumption. However, if we use less energy than we manufacture, we may notice a weight gain. If molecules of energy are not used, they turn to fat. To get rid of built up fat, more energy usually in the shape of exercise must be used or less energy through food taken in.

Basal Metabolism Rate (BMR)

This is the amount of energy required to keep the body alive when it is warm and at complete rest. It is used to keep the heart, lungs and digestive system moving. Women tend to have a lower BMR than men because they are lighter and have less muscle tissue. The BMR is also lower in elderly people and during periods of starvations, when the body needs lower food energy. The average values of BMR for person aged 40 year are:

Women: 1360 kcal (5700 kj) per day.
Men: 1750 kcal (7300 kj) per day.

Table below illustrates the energy used for various activities by a 25 year old male person weighing approximately 62 kg.

Activity	Kcal used/hour	Kj used/hour
Sleeping	57	238
Sitting	66	300
Standing	126	540
Washing/dressing	126	540
Walking moderately	210	900
Climbing stairs	390	1620
Dancing	270	1140
Jogging	390	1620

Seek advice of a doctor in the case of following conditions:

- If the age is under 18 or above 70 years.
- If undergoing medical treatment.
- In case of severe obesity.

- In case of a medical prescribed diet.
- In case of pregnancy or feeding a child.

Dietary advice for weight loss

- Combine a diet with an exercise program.
- Aim for a small, steady weight loss of ½ to 1 kilogram per week.
- Avoid crash diets.
- Other than a reduction in energy content, the diet must be well balanced.
- Eat three meals a day, so that the energy intake is spread evenly.
- Try to avoid eating in between meals.
- Drink plenty of fluids.

The Human organism

The human organism is made up of a vast variety of parts that vary in complexity. This include organs, tissue and cells. The cell is the basic structure from which all other body structures are made. These are the basic units of all living things including bacteria, plants and animals. The human body is composed entirely of cells, fluid and cellular products. Cells are made up of protoplasm—a colourless, jelly-like substance in which food elements such as protein, fats, carbohydrates, mineral salts and water are present. Cells have the following parts:

- **Cytoplasm:** Found outside the nucleus and contain materials necessary for the growth, reproduction and self-repair of the cell.
- **Centrosome:** A small round body in the cytoplasm, which also affects the reproduction of the cell.
- **Nucleus:** A small spherical body composed mostly of ribonucleic acid (RNA) and the protein within the cell nucleus. It plays an important part in the reproduction of the cell.
- **Cell membrane:** It encloses the protoplasm and permits soluble substance to enter and leave the cell.

The Cells, Body Tissue and Organs

In a human body, cell is a minute part that makes up each of the individual systems. The body is made up of millions of individual tiny microscopic cells. They are built into tissues, organs and glands, body systems and finally, the human organism. The cells varying in size and shape are made of protoplasm—a colourless, transparent, jelly-like substance consisting of nearly 70% water together with organic and inorganic substances.

Growth of a cell: As long as the cell receives an adequate supply of food, oxygen and water, eliminates waste products and is favoured with proper temperature, it will continue to grow and thrive. However, in case these conditions do not exist and there is the presence of toxins (poisons) or pressure, then the growth and the health of the cells are impaired. When the cells reaches maturity, reproduction takes place by direct or indirect division.

- **Direct division (Amitosis):** is a simple process whereby the cell elongates. This method of reproduction occurs among bacteria and plant life but rarely takes place in human tissues.
- **Indirect division (Mitosis):** is a complex process whereby a series of changes occur in the nucleus and this method of reproduction occurs in human tissues.

Body Tissues and Organs

Tissues are composed of group of cells. Each tissue has a specific function and can be recognized by its characteristic appearance. They are of five types:

- **Connective tissue:** Also known as fat tissues. They serve to support, protect and bind together tissues of the body.
- **Muscular tissue:** Contracts and move various parts of the body.
- **Nerve tissue:** Controls and coordinate all body functions.

- **Epithelial tissue:** A protective covering on the body surface such as skin, mucous, membranes, linings of heart, digestive and respiratory organs and glands.
- **Liquid tissue:** Carry food, waste products and hormones by means of the blood and lymph.

Organs

These are structures designed to accomplish a definite function. The important organs of the body are:

- **The brain:** Which controls the body.
- **The heart:** Which circulates the blood.
- **The lungs:** Which supply oxygen to the blood and controls respiratory system.
- **The liver:** Which removes toxic products of digestion.
- **The kidneys:** Which excrete water and other waste products.
- **The stomach and intestines:** Which helps to digest the food.

Recommended Dietary Allowance (RDA)

It is the daily requirement of nutrients that your body needs as recommended by the Indian Council of Medical Research. The RDA suggested for Indian women with a moderate activity level is given with an explanation of the functions and sources of all the major nutrients. Before conception, a woman should consume approximately 1900-2200 kcal/day as her daily energy requirement. However, during pregnancy, the energy requirements are higher and a woman needs between 2200-2500 kcal/day. These requirements should be supplemented by a balanced combination of carbohydratyes (cereals like whole wheat, ragi, jowar and paraboiled rice), protein (pulses and legumes), vegetables (green leafy vegetables) and the fat. It is not about how much you eat but what you eat. You must follow below-mentioned tips:

- **Daily energy requirement:** You need to provide your body with 2200 to 2500 kcal of energy per day to keep your strength up.
- **Daily protein requirement:** 65 gm. Good sources of protein are pulses (kidney beans and gram), dairy products (milk, cheese and curd) and Soybean products (tofu and soy chunks).
- **Daily calcium requirement:** 1000 mg/day. It is necessary for the development of bones and teeth. Eat plenty of foods such as dairy products, soybean products, green leafy vegetables (spinach, mint and fresh coriander), and sesame seeds.
- **Daily iron requirement:** 38 mg/day. Iron is necessary for hemoglobin (production of red blood cell), which supplies oxygen to each cell of the human body. If neglected, you might become anemic. Foods such as dried beans (peas and lentils), cereals and pulses, dried fruits (raisins, dates and figs), dark green leafy vegetables (spinach, mint, fresh coriander, cauliflower, broccoli and pumpkin), sesame seeds, nuts and almond enrich your iron stores.
- **Daily folic acid requirement:** Daily requirement about 400 mcg. It is an essential vitamin required especially for pregnant women and for those want to conceive. It helps formation of blood. And its deficiency leads to anemia. Potatoes, green vegetables (especially cluster beans, spinach, peas, broccoli, beetroot and ladies finger), cereals and pulses, soybean products, nuts, almonds and sesame seeds are beneficial sources.
- **Daily fat requirement:** It is a concentrated source of energy and a daily requirement of 30 gm of fat is essential.
- **Daily iodine requirement:** It is one of the major important minerals. To maintain adequate iodine level in your body, use iodized salt in your daily cooking.
- **Daily beta-Carotene (vitamin A) requirement:** Daily requirement 2400 mcg. It helps a healthy skin and cures skin disorders. Excessive Vitamin A can,

however, lead to toxicity and can be harmful. It is usually not necessary to supplement your diet with any other form of Vitamin A. Foods beneficial to increase Vitamin A are orange, vegetables (carrot, tomatoes and pumpkin), fruits (mango and papaya), dark green leafy vegetables (spinach, mint and fenugreek) and whole milk.

- **Daily vitamin C requirement:** Daily requirement 40 mg. It is required for the formation of collagen, make yourself immune against infections and diseases, to provide structure to the bones, cartilage, muscles and blood vessels.). Boost your Vitamin C levels with citrus fruits (orange, sweet lime and lemon), amla, vegetables (cabbage, coriander leaves and capsicum, fruit bean salad).
- **Daily vitamin D requirement:** Sunlight is the biggest source of vitamin D, which aids absorption of calcium in the body. Hence there is no dietary recommendation for this vitamin.
- **Daily requirement of vitamin B 12:** In comparison to non-vegetarian diets, vegetarian foods are deficient in vitamin B 12. Soymilk and other soy products provide maximum amount of this vitamin.

Few Precautions

- Buy fresh fruits and vegetables from the market. Seasonal fruits are the most nutritious.
- Refrigerating food for long periods results in the loss of vital nutrients. So always buy in small quantity and only that much quantity which is finished the same day.
- Eat vegetables and fruits without peeling so that your body receives full amount of fiber and nutrients. However, scrub these vegetables thoroughly before cooking as they may contain a thin of mud and pesticides.

- Do not soak vegetables in the water for a long time. It will make them lose many valuable, water-soluble vitamins such as vitamin B and vitamin C.
- Cook vegetables carefully so that they retain most of their nutrients during the cooking process. It is better to prepare vegetables by steaming process to retain most of the nutrients.
- In case you want to boil vegetables, use minimum quantity of water and cook only until the vegetable becomes tender.
- As far as possible, cook vegetables in large pieces as vegetable cut into small pieces lose more nutrients.
- Cover the foods while cooking to preserve the volatile nutrients present in vegetables and fruits.
- Prepare fresh salad or 'raita' before taking meals. Squeeze lemon on salads as it contains ample quantity of vitamin C, which helps in the absorption of iron from your meal.
- Include large amount of sprouts in your diet as sprouting aids in easy digestion. Sprouting destroys the anti-nutritional factors like phytates that are present in all legumes. They are called anti-nutritional factors because they hamper the absorption of vital nutrients like iron and calcium from the food. Sprouted peas and sprouted green gram are excellent source of vitamin C.
- Avoid using soda bicarbonate while cooking as it destroys most of the essential nutrients present in the food.

Diet while breastfeeding: While breastfeeding, a woman needs lot more calories than during the pregnancy period. Breastfeeding will make a woman burn 3500 kcal per day. However, she needs to consume only 2400 to 2700 kcal per day during the initial six months of lactation. During breastfeeding, stay off the ghee-laden dishes and try to have balanced diet and ensure that you have at least four liters of fluid every day. The following diet is required during lactating period:

Protein requirement: During the first six months of lactation 75 gm/day. Thereafter, reduce to 68 gm/day.

Fat:	45 gm/day
Calcium:	1000 mg/day
Iron:	30 mg/day
Folic acid:	150 mcg/day
Vitamin C:	80 mg/day
Vitamin A:	3800 mcg/day
Vitamin D:	There is no limitation as it aids the absorption of calcium in body
Other nutrients:	Your diet should include almonds, garlic, milk and fenugreek as all these products stimulate the production of breast milk.

Cholesterol and Premature Ageing

Cholesterol is a fatty substance that sticks to the insides of our blood vessels and make them narrower, enabling heart to pump harder in order to get youth-enhancing nutrients.

If the excess builds up on artery walls, it can clog your arteries and restrict blood flow, possibly leading to a heart attack, stroke or angina pain. When your cholesterol levels are high, you have got too much of a mushy, yellow, fat-related substance circulating in the bloodstream. Blood also performs some pretty vital job and helps to build new cells, produce hormones and insulate nerves. The ratio between good and bad cholesterol is very important. The more overweight you are, the more cholesterol your body produces. The chart below gives the total cholesterol level according to age in both sexes.

Age	Total cholesterol level in men	Total cholesterol level in women
Under 30	179	179
30-39	191	186
40-49	205	194
50-59	208	219
60 +	208	221

Ways to Stay Cholesterol on the Lower Side

- Large doses of niacin, also known as nicotinic acid helps to lower both high-density lipoprotein (HDL) cholesterol and low-density lipoprotein (LDL). It is better to start off with low doses (up to 100 mg a day) and gradually increase to 1 or 2 gm a day over a period of several weeks. Remember, sudden increases in niacin can produce severe overall flushing, intestinal disorders and sometimes abnormal liver function. Better seek advice of your doctor.
- Vitamin C when added to a pectin-rich diet, cholesterol level drops. Many pectin packed fruits and vegetables such as citrus fruit, tomatoes, potatoes, strawberries and spinach are rich in vitamin C. Vitamin E is useful for people with mildly high levels of cholesterol. 500 international units of vitamin E a day for 90 days increases HDL level.
- Calcium supplements for the sake of your bones. 1 gm of calcium daily for eight weeks lowers cholesterol level by 4.8%, whereas 2 gm of calcium carbonate a day reduces cholesterol level by 25% in a year.
- Watch your weight carefully. A diet composed of two-third fruits, vegetables, cereals and whole grains controls your cholesterol level. Only one-third of your calories should come from meat and dairy products.
- Cut the fat. Three principal dietary factors have an impact on blood cholesterol levels. Saturated fat elevates blood cholesterol. Polyunsaturated fat lowers blood cholesterol. The third one Dietary cholesterol contributes to elevated blood cholesterol to a lesser degree than saturated fat and poly-unsaturated fat. So it is wise to cut sources of fat such as meat, butter, cheese and hydrogenated oil. As far as possible, replace these items with fish, poultry, low-fat dairy products and oils such as corn, safflower and soybean. Switch to olive oil, which may lower cholesterol level.

- Exercise decreases the build up of cholesterol blockage inside the arteries. Exercise increases the body's ability to clear fat from the blood.
- Garlic and onions can reduce harmful blood fats.

What is Antioxidant?

If a free radical is a fire, an oxidant is a bucket full of water to control fire. Oxygen gives both life and death. An antioxidant is a substance that prevents damage as a result of oxygen reactions or oxidation. Oxygen reactions throw off destructive free radicals, Antioxidants neutralize the damage done by the radicals. Our bodies have a natural defense system consisting of certain enzymes. The most powerful internal free radical fighters is an enzyme called super-oxide dismutage. The prominent anti-oxidants are: vitamin C, vitamin E, beta carotene and calcium, which exist inside certain foods, and we eat these foods, we release the antioxidants.

Antioxidant and Longevity

- People who take vitamins, especially antioxidant, live longer than people who do not.
- Antioxidants boost ageing immune system, rejuvenate them and make them strong to fight off killer attacks from pneumonia, bacteria, viruses and other invaders.
- Antioxidants can slow and in some cases even reverse the growth of cancer cells.
- Antioxidants can clean out clogged arteries, lower cholesterol levels and reduce the risk of heart attacks, stroke and hypertension.
- Antioxidants can help bones remain strong and restore lost bone tissue.
- Antioxidant can smooth wrinkles, reduce fine lines, crow's feet, fade age spots an strengthen and rejuvenate collagen.
- Antioxidants can restore vision.
- Antioxidant can help prevent senility, diseases of nervous system and premature loss of brain functions.

- Antioxidants protect against damage from environment pollutants like cigarette smoke, exhaust fumes and chemical sprays.
- Antioxidants can help you shed weight.
- And the list goes on, and on, and on.

The recommended Dietary Allowances are levels of intake of essential nutrients considered. The RDA for antioxidants is set in such a way as to prevent disease from a serious deficiency. However, RDAs are not set to take into account special needs such as the fighting of infections, strenuous exercise, chronic illness or injury. According to the experts, it is safe to get more than the RDA for antioxidants. Most of the experts now recommend a longevity dose of antioxidant protection.

Antioxidant Dosages: a Comparison

Antioxidant	RDA	Longevity doses
Vitamin C	60 mg	800-1000 mg
Beta-carotene	50 IU	10,000 IU
Vitamin E	30 IU	400-800 IU
Calcium	1000 mg	1000-1500 mg

Vitamin C-capsule to Remain Young

Vitamin C is a water-soluble carbohydrate. It is a powerful anti-ageing weapon having the following benefits:

- Keeps complexion wrinkle-free.
- Make hips and thighs smooth without ugly bumps and dimples of cellulite.
- Helps to keep bones straight, tall and slender.
- Vitamin C plays a role in the manufacture of serotonin—the potent brain chemical that can help lose weight. We can boost serotonin simply by eating right amount of carbohydrates in combination with other foods. This helps to restore energy, end emotional overeating and control weight increase. According to a medical research, 300 mg of vitamin C

a day adds six years to a man's life and two years to a woman's life. Another study found that vitamin C can actually reverse aging by rejuvenating white blood cells—giving 76 year olds the same look as 30 year olds, if only 120 mg of vitamin C a day or one and half cups of fresh strawberries is taken daily.

- Protects skin from ultraviolet damage leading to wrinkles. A study reveals that vitamin C can make a real difference in protecting exposed skin from the damage caused by the sun, environmental pollutants, and even cigarette smoking. The vitamin C youth capsules helps in fewer lines and wrinkles, less skin cancer, and a more youthful, dewy complexion.
- Men with high level of vitamin C in their systems are less likely to die from heart disease, especially when they have a diet rich in vitamin C.
- According to National Cancer Institute, vitamin C works like a antibiotic against viruses that attack and weaken our immune system and also triggers the production of interferon, which is one of our body's natural defenses against foreign invaders that can damage and destroy our healthy living cells and tissue.
- Vitamin C reduces risk of developing lung problems like asthma, chronic bronchitis and other disorders.

The Recommended Dietary Allowance of Vitamin C

Pregnant women:	80 mg
Lactating women:	100 mg
Infants from birth to 6 months:	35 mg
Infants from 6 to 12 months:	35 mg
Children from 1 to 10 years:	45 mg
Children from 11 to 18 years:	50 mg
Adults:	60 mg
Heavy smokers	100 mg

Vitamin C Supplements

Most experts agree that vitamin C is most effective when it comes from food sources because it comes in little packages with other vital anti-ageing nutrients. Following are top food sources of vitamin C:

- **Fruits:** Papaya, Guava, Strawberries, Orange, Mango, Lemon, Grapefruit, Mandarin orange, Honeydew melon, Pineapple, Watermelon, Blackberries, Banana, Apricot and Grape.
- **Vegetables:** Pepper, Brussels sprouts, Peas, Sweet potato, Cauliflower, Broccoli,, Kale, Parsley, Collards, Onions, Cabbage, Tomato, Beet greens, Mustard greens, Soybeans, Spinach, Asparagus, Spinach, Avocado and Radish.
- **Juices:** Orange, Lemon, Cranberry, Grapefruit, Lime, Tomato and Pineapple.

Vitamin E: a Miraculous Fat Buster Vitamin

Benjamin Franklin rightly said that one should eat to live, not live to eat. It works to protect the fatty parts of our cells and fight to knock out free radicals in human body.

It is vitamin E that is credited with projecting the fragile immune cell membranes, which are defensive to fight diseases, pump nutrients-rich blood to every part of body, keep heart and other organs of body working, increase the average life span and premature ageing, protect our delicate cells from the damage and destruction of sunshine. Vitamin E regulates brain cells that control anti-ageing mechanism in the body.

How Vitamin E Slows Overall Ageing?

Vitamin E scrubs ageing pigments from our body cells, which are known as lipofuscin—rusty brown sludge that shows up as age spots on our skin, internal organs and damage brain cells, which cause cellular destruction and ultimately premature ageing or death. A research reveals that men and women who take 100 to 250 IU of vitamin E, as advised by the doctor, reduces the risk of heart attack and other cardiovascular and lung problems by approximately 40%. Vitamin E helps to boost immune system that inhibits the growth and spread of cancer cells in the body, relieve arthritis, develop cataracts, cure dreaded brain disease Alzheimer and protect the skin from the more visible signs of ageing such as fine lines, wrinkles, age spots, protect against the development and growth of deadly skin cancers when taken internally.

How Much Vitamin E is Enough?

Research points that most of the people get enough vitamin E from our daily diet, which offers minimum protection. However, longevity experts agree that average RDA obtainable from daily diet ranging between 12 to 15 IU is not enough. So most recommended amount of this vitamin for an adult should amount to between 100 to 400 IU a day for men and women, as advised by a doctor. Remember, vitamin E is fat soluble, and is amply found in polyunsaturated fats such as vegetable oils. These add unwanted fat calories to the diet. The best food sources of vitamin E are listed below:

Food	Serving	Vitamin E (IU)
Wheat germ oil	1 tablespoon	25
Sunflower seeds	1 ounce	21
Almonds	1 ounce	11
Sunflower oil	1 tablespoon	10
Safflower oil	1 tablespoon	8
Wheat germ	1 ounce	5
Margarine	1 tablespoon	3
Rice brown	1 cup	3
Peanut (dry, roasted)	1 ounce	3
Mango	1 medium	3
Avocado	1 medium	3
Soybean oil	1 tablespoon	2
Spinach	1 cup	1

As far as possible, take your vitamin E supplement last thing at bedtime along with your calcium supplement.

Beta-carotene: Vitamin A is Anti-aging Dose

You will like to know the difference between beta-carotene and vitamin A. Beta-carotene is what we get when we eat bright green, yellow, red and orange fruits and vegetables. After the beta-carotene is swallowed, it travels through the digestive system and reaches the intestine and turns into vitamin A. Beta-carotene helps to beat wrinkles and restore smooth, line-free, youthful skin. It restores self-esteem and reduces the stress of visible aging.

Recommended Dietary Allowances of Vitamin A

Age	Dietary allowance in IU
1-5 months	4200
6 months-3 years	4000
4 years-6 years	5000
7 years-10 years	7000
Adult males	10,000
Adult females	8000
Pregnant women	10,000
Nursing mothers	12,000

Food Sources of Beta-Carotene

- Fruits and vegetables: Apricots (dried or fresh), Beet greens, Broccoli, Carrots, dandelion greens, Endive, Garden cress, Kale, Lettuce, Mango, Muskmelon, Papaya, Parsley, Peppers, Peas, Pumpkin, Spinach and Sweet potato.
- Chicken liver, Chicken giblets, Turkey soup, Chicken soup and milk.

Calcium: Adds Years to Your Age

Lack of calcium may cause:

- Prematurely gray hair.
- Sticking out tummy.
- Breast cancer.

- High blood pressure.
- Dental problems.

If the answer to any of them is Yes, you are definitely not getting enough calcium. A calcium deficiency can sabotage your weight loss, your posture, your energy level and even your sexy smile. Nearly 98% of the calcium in our body is stored in skinny storage units called bones and the remaining 2% circulates throughout our bodies carried in the bloodstream. As an antioxidant mineral, calcium blocks the oxygen starvation leading to diminished bone mass, protects cell membranes from destruction by free radicals, regulates the level of calcium in blood and bones and relieves all premature ageing diseases. A survey reveals that most women die of osteoporosis starting around the age 30 than of breast cancer, cancer of the cervix and the cancer of the uterus combined. Doctors recommend a low-fat diet and at least 1000 mg of calcium a day from a combination of food and supplements. It helps to cure blood pressure and colon cancer.

Recommended Daily Calcium Diet

Age and status	Mg per day
Infants from birth to 6 months	400
Infants from 6 months to 1 year	600
Children from 1 to 5 years	800
Children from 6 to 10 years	800-1200
Adolescents from 11 to 24 years	1200 to 1500
Pregnant adolescents	2000
Pregnant women	1200 to 1500
Pre-menopausal women 25-40 years	1000
Post-menopausal women on estrogen	1000
Post-menopausal women not on estrogen	1500
Men 25 to 65 years	1000
Men above 65 years	1500

Calcium Robbers

Salt, caffeine, fatness, excessive intake of protein, smoking and alcohol are biggest enemies of calcium. A medical report confirms that 2600 mg of sodium can wipe out 891 mg of calcium. There is no risk to calcium if three cups of coffee are taken in a day with the addition of a little skim milk to each cup. Remember, coffee is not the only caffeine culprit, even hot tea, chocolate and colas harm due to caffeine contents in it.

Fat can combine with calcium and convert it to a form that cannot be absorbed by the body resulting in we get fatter but our bones get thinner. Human body do need protein, but not too much of it. Smoking is harmful and creates lot of free radicals that attack calcium stored in bones and destroy delicate bone tissue, thus cause premature ageing.

Little quantity of alcohol may be good for your bones, raise estrogen levels in the body, protect the heart and lowers blood pressure. But too much of alcohol is harmful for the body, sucks calcium out of bones and weaken them. 1200 mg to 1500 mg calcium taken every day is an excellent anti-ageing dose.

Top Food Sources of Calcium

Foods	Calcium contents in mg
Spinach, fresh, ½ cup cooked	122
Turnip greens, fresh, 1/s cup cooked	99
Kale, frozen, ½ cup cooked	90
Broccoli, fresh, ½ cup cooked	89
Mustard greens, frozen, ½ cup cooked	75
Orange 1 medium size	52
Tomato juice, 1 cup	22
Carrot, 1 of medium size	19
Raisins, ¼ cup	18
Milk, skim, 1 cup	302
Buttermilk, 1 cup	285
Ice cream, ½ cup	118
Yogurt, plain non-fat, 1 cup	452
Cheese, 1 ounce	355

7

Self-health Care to Control Ageing

Daily care of your health and beauty ensure that the natural beauty of your body does not fade away too soon and you remain young for long. Here are few basic guidelines for self-care of your health, beauty and body regime a woman can maintain during early, middle, menopausal period, the period of pregnancy and post-natal. Today, when women become pregnant, they look forward to a birth that is not only safe but also satisfying. When you are pregnant, it's important to be aware of the effect your changing weight is having on your posture and to adjust it accordingly to maintain a state of harmonious balance. It is often seen that after childbirth, women loose the shape of their body and look ten year older. Good posture should be dynamic, alive and always changing according to your needs.

Childbirth

Childbirth is a natural process, even when it comes unexpectedly at home or on the way to the hospital. If you are in labour or with someone who is about to give birth, don't try to stop the process or delay delivery. Stay calm and call the doctor. The expectant mother has the following symptoms:

- Contraction of uterus two to three minutes apart.
- A vaginal discharge.

- An overwhelming urge by the woman to push, or to move her bowel.
- Feeling or seeing the baby's head to emerge.

Under these circumstances, go to the emergency room right away. If there is no time to get to a hospital, prepare a place with plastic sheet and clean linens and pillow. Keep the expectant woman comfortable as much as possible. Help her to take off her clothes from the waist down. Try to get an aged lady to advise the operation till the arrival of doctor or midwife. There will be some bloody fluid and other discharge. Watch for the baby's head to appear in the opening to the vagina. Be ready to support baby's head as it comes through the vagina. Baby's shoulders and body should follow on the next contractions. Do not pull the baby's head; support it gently as the shoulders slide out. When the head emerges, watch for umbilical cord wrapped around the baby's neck: ease

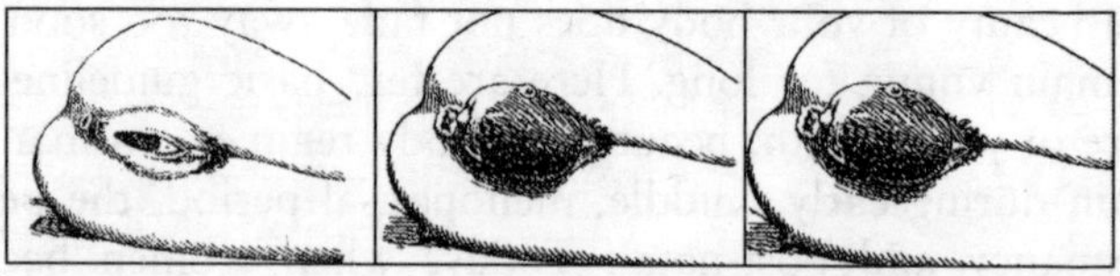

it over the baby's head with two fingers. There may be gush of fluid when the baby's body slides out and the baby will be very slippery. If the baby doesn't come out headfirst, do not try to pull the baby out; support as best as you can and expose the face so that the baby can breathe. Do not cut the umbilical cord; and wait for the doctor to do it. Wipe baby's nose and mouth gently with a clean cloth to remove mucus and other fluids so that they do not get into the baby's lungs.

Posture Problem During Pregnancy

When you are pregnant, it's important to be aware of the effect your changing weight is having on your posture and to adjust it accordingly to maintain a state of harmonious balance. The rocking movements and small adjustments mentioned below are aimed at helping you find your centre of balance from early months of pregnancy until the last few weeks. To achieve good posture:

- Stand with your feet hip-width apart, so that your legs fall straight down from the hip joints.
- Have your feet in line with one another, turning outward no more than a fraction.
- Rock back and forth between the heels and the balls of your feet to find the central point at which your weight is well balanced over the whole of each foot. Make sure the arches remain lifted, so that you are not rolling your feet either inward or outward.
- Bend your knees very slightly, so that they are at ease.
- Rock your pelvis by tilting your pubic bone forward and back a few times to find the mid-point. Remember, the pelvis is the heaviest part of the body and your centre of gravity. Make sure, it is centred properly. Check that you are not twisting it by holding one hip slightly farther forward than the other.
- Lift your ribs up as far from your hips as you can, so that your chest opens out, your shoulders drop down and the back and your arms roll slightly outward. Drop your ribs and lift arms again a few times.
- Pull your shoulders down away from your ears and at the same time lengthen the back of your neck upward.
- Balance your head with the chin at about a right angle to the front of your neck.

The Benefits of Good Posture During and After Pregnancy

- Your ribs and chest lift, so you can expand the rib cage and breathe well.
- Your abdominal muscles are not allowed to sag, so they act as a strong corset. Therefore, support the growing weight and soon regain the original shape after the birth.
- The pelvis is correctly positioned, so both the buttocks and abdomen help support the trunk, and prevent lower back strain.

- The back of the neck lengthens upward, so your head is well balanced and doesn't compress your neck or distort your spine.
- Your shoulders are dropped, thus preventing unnecessary tension in the shoulders, neck and the upper back.
- Your spine is lengthened, which allow plenty of space to your baby in womb.

Effect of hormones and the posture: The changes in the menstrual cycle usually occur due to female sex hormones from the regulating centre—the pituitary gland influenced by the brain. The pituitary glands stimulate the ovaries to secrete estrogen hormones. The ovaries begin the secretion of progesterone for the preparation of fertilized egg to get settled in the uterus. There is sudden drop in the level of progesterone and estrogen, the inner lining of uterus starts breaking up and escapes out through vagina mixed with blood as menstrual flow. This changing cycle leaves adverse effect on a woman's posture.

Pigmentation of skin cause premature ageing: Pigmentation on the facial skin is a major problem during periods. What we want is an even toned, translucent, radiant and blemish-free skin and slim-trim body during these days. The melanin in the skin is the culprit. The amount and distribution of this pigment determines skin colour and differs. The imbalance in the amount and distribution stay on just the upper layer of the skin or run deep as well. Hyper-pigmentation is usually faced by women during periods, pregnancy and post-natal. The common problems related to pigmentation are Melasma: a brownish discolouration that usually starts after pregnancy, usually seen on the face (cheeks, forehead and nose) and other parts on the body, but tends to persist till the delivery of infant and lactating period. There are several treatments available, to cope with pigmentation and your posture, you can select one according to the recommendation of your doctor.

How to Control Ageing During Pregnancy?

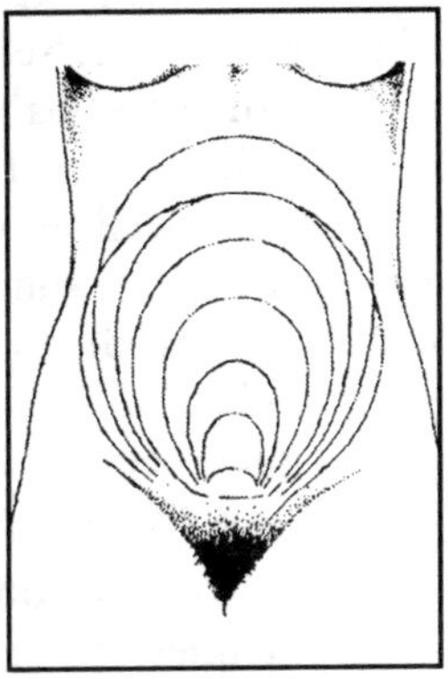

Pregnancy can change your appearance due to rapid hormonal changes, which cause dry, flaky skin or a blotchy acne-prone complexion. Body undergoes many changes including severe fatness during pregnancy. Skin is the first thing to bear the burn of it. Some of the common problems include very dry, itchy skin, melasma, acne and stretch marks. Do not despair as these can be treated during and after pregnancy. Usually, from the second trimester of pregnancy, a pregnant woman might suddenly find herself with very dry, taut skin that is sand papery to the touch, especially around the stomach, breasts, hands and legs. Avoid worrying, generally the condition vanishes after delivery. But till then, be sure to keep skin extra moisturized with a creamy body lotion. Almond oil or cocoa butter based creams tend to work wonders in soothing the skin during this period when applied after bath.

Stretch Marks on Face and Body During Pregnancy

For most women, the skin tends to clear up during pregnancy due to extra blood flow in the system. Few women give rise to acne and pimples. Stretch marks are undoubtedly the biggest problem that almost all pregnant women worry about. This happens when the skin loses its elasticity due to the stretching of the upper and lower layers of the skin. They generally appear as red marks, which form white strip-like marks across stomach. With timely treatment and massage with vitamin E oil accompanied by a balanced diet, the stretch marks may lighten.

Care Taken During the First three Months of Pregnancy

Pregnancy can also be a time of difficulty for a mother-to-be. There are additional physical strains to cope with along with confusing and conflicting advice from friends and relatives. In the midst of such pressures, a pregnant woman often has no time for her beauty and body care. But it is very important for an expectant woman to spend some of her time thinking about herself. If the expectant mother is relaxed and healthy, then her baby stands a good chance of being healthy too. The 40 weeks of pregnancy have several beauty and body problems as well as some beauty bonuses. Nature may prove very good for some mother-to-be. They may find that pregnancy produces unexpected benefits like clear skin, glowing cheeks, glossy hair and attractive body. An expectant mother may become beautiful, if she starts taking extra beauty care from the very beginning as detailed below:

- **How to look after your body?:** During the first trimester of pregnancy, there is great hormonal activity in the body. The figure becomes aged, plump and lumpy. The joy of realizing that you are going to be a mother may be clouded by doubts and disappointment over the way you look disfigured.

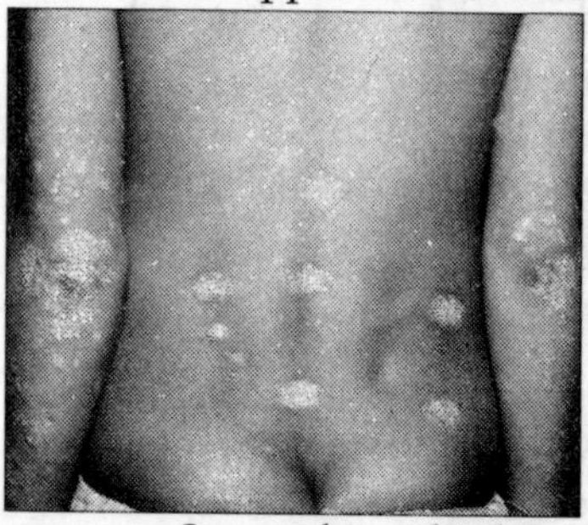

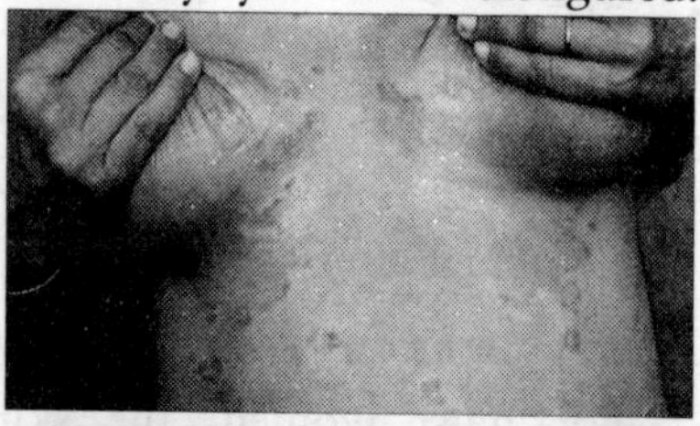

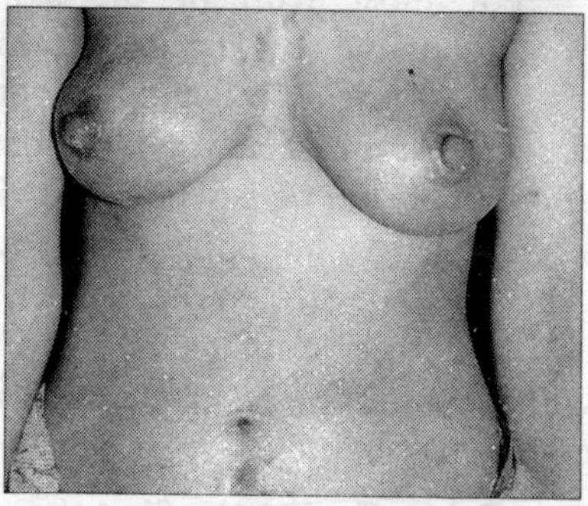

Start by thinking positive about your beauty care and a daily beauty routine. Spots appearing on the face, chest or back should not worry you as the increased hormonal activity in your body is causing this temporary upset. Never squeeze any spot anywhere on your body to get rid of it, which may leave a permanent scar. When you are pregnant, pay special attention to lubricate the skin on your stomach, buttocks and breasts. Apply plenty of skin conditioning cream after your bath and rub in baby oil or olive oil every night. Stretch marks are very difficult to remove after the birth of baby. Lubrication of the skin at this time can prevent spots and wrinkles and pay handsome dividend later on. Keep lubricating throughout the nine months of pregnancy period.

- **Diet control:** You need more attention on your diet in this period. You need more nutrients, not more calories. Cut out fried, sweet and fatty foods. If you are non-vegetarian, fish provides Vitamin D, which you need at this stage. Drink a glass of milk a day, it fulfils the need of Calcium. Take smaller meals more frequently during the day. Avoid really strenuous exercise during the crucial first three months. Go to the bed early. The most radiant mother-to-be of all is the rested one.

Care taken During Second Trimester

Beauty and body care taken early in pregnancy now begins to pay dividends. Hair and skin conditions improve at this stage. The following steps should be taken:

- Continue with daily stomach, bottom and breast lubrication and pay special attention to skin freshness.
- Underarm depilation and deodorizing are essential.
- Night cramps are often a problem at this stage. Massage your legs before sleep.
- Keep strict watch on your diet and weight gain. Total weight gain during pregnancy should be about 12 kg. Remember, toxaemia (blood poisoning) and high blood pressure are dangers for overweight mothers-to-be, and so are varicose veins.
- Keep walking with your doctor's advice. Walk slowly. It is important to keep up light exercise as per your doctor's approval.

- Going to bed early during this period is a good habit to enhance body grooming.
- The most comfortable position in bed is lying on your side with one leg slightly in front of the other, one hand under the pillow, and the other by your side. That way the weight is evenly distributed.

Care taken During the Final Months

This is the time for the final preparations to welcome the baby. Take good care of you ,as you need a lot of energy in the coming months to bring up baby as well as to retain your beauty and posture. Take the following steps:

- Dryness and blotchiness are sometimes problems at the end of pregnancy period. Take care to nourish your skin rightly. Give your body plenty of skin cream in the last two months.
- If you intend to breastfeed your baby, keep your nipples soft with a special cream to help prevent cracking and massage breasts to avoid over-development and fat.
- Increase milk and high protein food in your diet. Keep your iron intake high, too. Drink fresh orange juice instead of tea or coffee. A high Vitamin C intake helps protect you against infections.
- When labour begins, have a good meal.
- A good sleep is necessary during the final month.

Post-natal Care of Your Beauty and Body

Having a baby takes a great deal of energy. Even though you have been following a good anti-natal beauty program, you are bound to feel tired and exhausted for first few months after the birth of child. The following care should be taken:

- Make sure that your diet is rich in nutrients such as plenty of vitamin C, protein and minerals. Keep up the iron supplement you took before baby was born.

- Take care of your body and have regular exercise, otherwise you will loose shape of your body and look aged.

The Pelvis

Before becoming pregnant for the first time, many women are surprisingly unaware of the internal workings of their own bodies. However, once the pregnancy is confirmed, the pelvis and its associated muscles and organs become the centre of interest and it is important to understand the role of the pelvis in pregnancy and childbirth. The bones of the pelvis form the strong frame that acts like a cradle, surrounding, supporting and protecting the womb.

The pelvic floor is the essential sling of muscle that helps to hold the pelvic organs in place. Several layers deep, the pelvic muscles are slung under the pelvis in two intersecting circles, which look like a figure 'Eight (8)'. The larger, top ring of the muscle controls the outlets of the urethral and vaginal sphincters. Below is the smaller circle of muscle, which contains the stronger anal or rectal, sphincter. The muscles overlap and so they are thicker at the perineum, the area between the anus and vagina.

Pelvic floor exercises are important throughout your life. Sensitivity in this area increases your love making enjoyment. If the muscles become slack you will find that you lack enjoy during sexual intercourse as much and may have difficulty reaching orgasm. Your male partner will also find love making less enjoyable. Remember, a weak pelvic floor can lead to incontinence and even prolapse, and sagging of the walls of the vagina besides losing the shape of your body.

Take Care to Practice the Following Pelvis Exercises

The following movements will help you prepare the pelvic area for childbirth. Practice these movements daily in rhythmic slow motion, repeating each for five to six times. These simple exercises will help provide you the best position for shaping your body and help a painless delivery.

- **Pelvic tilt (standing position):** The pelvic tilt by lifting pubic bone up in the front is an essential movement for maintaining good posture during pregnancy and after the birth, support the trunk, strengthen abdominal and buttock muscles to minimize strain on the lower back. To do this exercise, stand with your feet little away from the wall, hip width apart, bend knees slightly and rest your back, shoulders and head against the wall. Breathe in. As you breathe out, press your lower back firmly against the wall, pulling in your abdomen and lifting your pubic bone, so your buttocks tighten and leave the wall. Keep shoulders pressed against the wall and move the pelvis only.

- **Pelvic tilt (second posture):** Kneel with your knees in line with your hips and hands in line with your shoulders. Keep your back flat. Now pull in your abdominal muscles, tighten your buttocks and do a pelvic tilt, so your back humps up. Do not rock your pubic bone back in this position or when lean forwards, that might strain your back.
- **Dancing exercise:** Dancing is an excellent exercise. Rocking and circling the pelvis are basic movements in all rhythmic dance. You may dance to music either standing or kneeling or on all fours circling the pelvis. The regular practice of this exercise helps comfort during labour.

Spine

The spine is the supporting structure of the body connecting your head, ribs, pelvis and limbs. Between each movable joint of the spine is a soft jelly-like disc that allows freedom of the movement. If you allow your spine to sag, these soft discs may become squashed causing stiffness and pain, and make you look sick and aged. Muscles of the back, too, help you to keep the spine lengthen. If your back is stiff and inflexible, loosen it up with the exercises as detailed in this chapter. Gently twisting your back is relaxing and invigorating and helps to prevent you straining. Stretch out your back with pelvic tilt before you start exercising. Spinal Exercises are the following:

- Stretch your spine sitting, standing or lying down. Practice the movement sitting against a wall. Pull your shoulder blades together and down. Then press your back against the wall, giving a pelvic tilt. Get into the habit of practising this movement whenever you settle into a chair or car seat.
- Sit against the wall pressing your back. Now stretch your arms above your head at the same time, flattening them as far back as you can against the wall. Keep your shoulders down.
- Kneel with your knees hip-width apart. Slowly twist to the right. Hold for a moment; then repeat to the left. Prevent twisting your hips and thighs.
- Sit cross-legged. Press against your knee to help you twist farther.
- Stand straight, both knees facing forward. Swing your arms for extra momentum and twist from side to side standing.

The spine massage: The spine is built of small bones called vertebrae, which are stacked in a column. Between the bones are spongy discs. The spinal cord is a bunch of nerve fibers running down a channel through the spine. Vertebrae are mounted on a solid base attached to the pelvis. Perform the following movements:

- Start massaging at the neck with index and middle fingers on either side of the spine.
- Make firm strokes downwards on the back simultaneously with both hands one after the other.
- Now place the right hand at the base of spine resting middle of the palm on the bone of the spinal cord and press the spine with middle finger. Avoid pressing hard on the vertebrae.
- Now apply stretching movement. Cross arms and place one hand on the sacrum and the other on the centre of the spinal cord with hands facing away from each other.

- Apply a diagonal stretch to the back placing one hand on the shoulder and other on the hip. After massaging for some time, repeat movement on the other shoulder.

How to Strengthen Your Back and Look Young?

Try to straighten your back, as the straightening motion strengthens the back muscles. 'Tailor sitting' has the following beneficial effects:

- Strengthens the muscles of back.
- Useful in preparation for labour as it loosens the groin and hips, and stretches the muscles of the inner thighs.
- Stimulates the circulation in the lower half of the body. Practising this will help you to hold a variety of positions in labour and will let your legs wide apart during the delivery of child.

The following is the procedure for Tailor sitting:

Sit on the floor with the soles of your feet together. Hold your ankles. Bring your pelvis and feet as close together as you can by walking forward on your hips. Keep your back straight. In case you feel uncomfortable in practising this posture, place a couple of cushions under each of your thighs for support.

You may practice this exercise in lying down position: You may try this posture in lying down position. Practice Tailor sit posture and lean backward slowly till your back touches the floor. You can seek the help of your partner while leaning backward, and coming to initial Tailor sitting position after few seconds.

Exercises to Strengthen Your Back

Sit against a wall to feel the length of your spine. Lift knees upward so that the soles of both feet press each other. This is also a good way to check whether your back is really straight. Sit straight without giving support of wall. Prop yourself up with your arms on the floor to help you lift. Make a loose fist with each hand and press the fist into the floor behind you as you lift your ribs away from the hips and straighten your back. Make sure that shoulders do not move up.

Sitting, Leg Apart for Slimming Lower Body

This exercise stretches the groin, inside thighs, back of the legs and strengthens the quadriceps—the muscles at the front

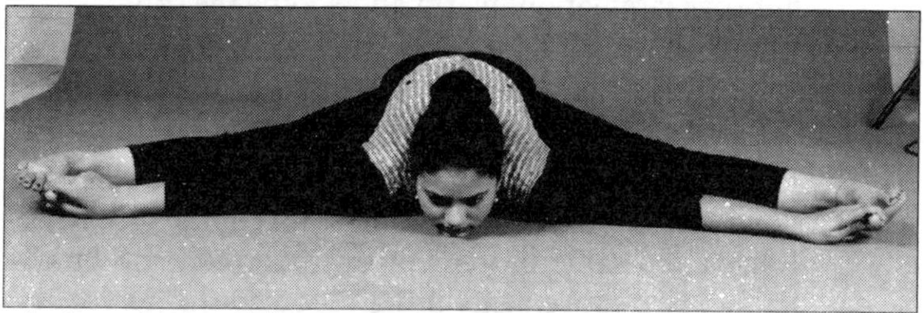

of the thighs. This exercise is particularly important in pregnancy when the extra weight can put undue strain on the knees. The exercise strengthens the muscles and also helps you to cope with the weight of the baby. To practice this exercise, sit straight, lifting your back. Wide your legs apart as much as you can sideways, one leg at a time. Tighten the muscles of your legs and keep toes pointing upwards. Now hook big toes with your index and middle fingers. If hands do not touch the feet, take them up to the point you do comfortably. Bend forward and rest your forehead or chin on the floor. If it is uncomfortable, do not practice this exercise. Do not bend your knees. This exercise has the following advantages:

- Improves circulation in the pelvic region and makes hamstring muscles elastic.
- Makes delivery easier and relieves labour pains.
- This exercise is especially good for women other than pregnant for curing all menstruation disorder.
- Strengthen genital organs and increases sex power.
- This exercise keeps joints, muscles, organs and nerves strong and healthy.
- Slim the body and make you look younger.

How to massage back?: The following steps are performed for massaging back:

- Put thumbs on either side of the spine. Stroke firmly up on the back till hands reach the shoulders (on the upper curves of shoulders).

- Glide the hands tightly downwards on both sides of the back till the hands reach the waist and the hips.
- Repeat movement 10 to 12 times daily. This will improve circulation, warm and soothe the skin.
- Stroke at the sides of the back with loose, relaxed hands. Now pull in towards the spine with one hand following the other in a smooth, flowing rhythm.
- Place both hands in one side on the back. Pressing downwards stroke both hands in circles clockwise. Repeat the same movement on the other side on the back. Brisk movements bring blood to the nerves and eases pain.

Breasts

Your breasts are likely to become larger and heavier during pregnancy, and unless you support them with a well-fitting bra, they may sag and lose their shape. So even if you don't normally wear a bra, you should do so while your breasts are heavy. There are no muscles in the breasts themselves, but you

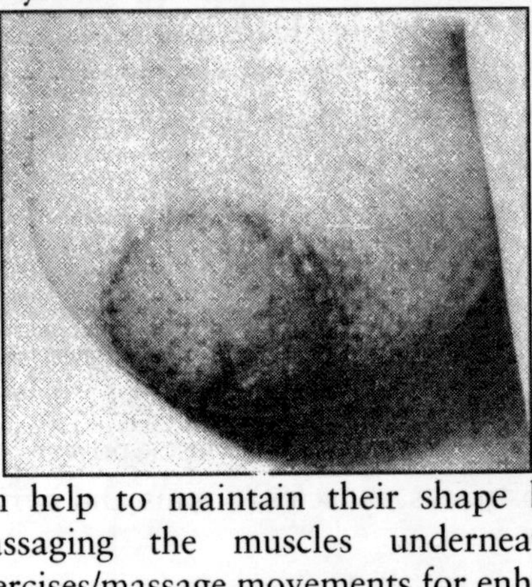

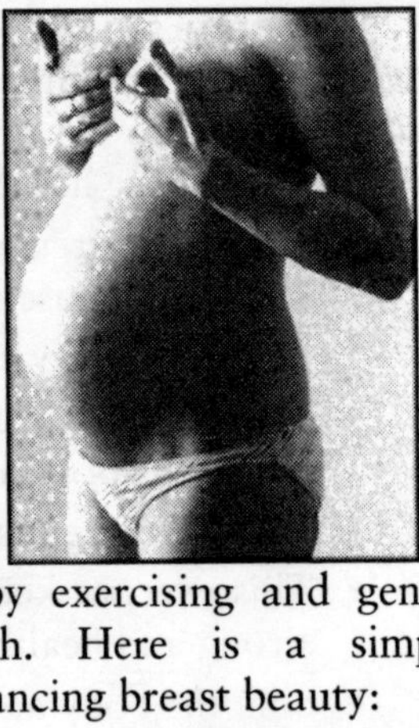

can help to maintain their shape by exercising and gently massaging the muscles underneath. Here is a simple exercises/massage movements for enhancing breast beauty:

- Make a loose fist with one hand and clasp the other round it. Hold your hands in level with your breasts and press together tightly for few moments. Repeat the sequence several times.

- Massage helps to re-shape your breasts which start expanding during pregnancy and become saggy and shapeless during post-natal when the baby feeds. A regular massage in the bathroom after shower or bath during pregnancy and when the mother is breastfeeding, the baby is very helpful to strengthen breast muscle. Start massage making slow, gentle strokes with both hands over the bulge.

Abdomen

Strong abdominal muscles help you carry the baby more easily without straining your back. They are also helpful during the birth, when the baby is being pushed out; better the condition of your abdomen muscles, the easier it is to restore them afterwards. The following exercises/massage movements help strengthening the abdominal muscles and fight aging:

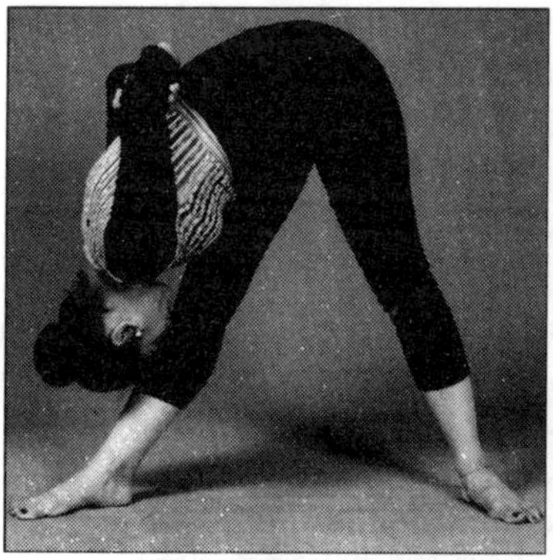

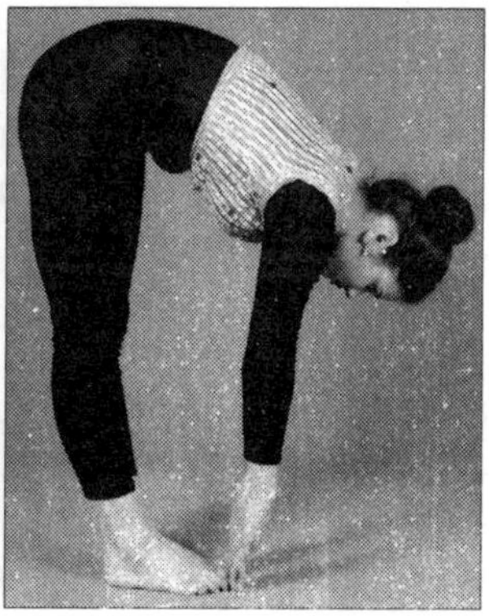

- The most important exercise for the abdomen muscles is simply to pull in your abdomen as you breathe out, as often as you can.
- Triangle Posture gets you rid of flab around the waist and abdomen. Stand with the legs apart. Rotate waist, begin to exhale until the fingers of the right hand touch the ground. Hold for some time, stand up and perform the same movement to the other hand. This posture makes the entire body strong and elastic, and also toning the muscles in the back, hips and legs.

- Sun Exercise is very helpful to remain young. Stand straight with arms on sides. Raise both arms upward, stretched. Inhale slowly, bend downward and touch the floor with both hands. This posture tones up the muscles of abdomen, waist, hips and relieve extra fat from these areas.
- Curl ups exercises are beneficial throughout pregnancy, except perhaps during the last few weeks, if you get very large. Continue curl ups movements as long as they are not uncomfortable. Just remember not to strain, if you feel pressure on the pelvic floor, the exercise is too strenuous. To practice this exercise, lie on your back with your legs bent, feet hip-width apart, your hands on your thighs. Breathe in. As you breathe out, raise your head and shoulders, dropping your chin and reaching towards your knees. Sometimes, your shoulders won't lift up smoothly for few days after the childbirth. Gradually, they will start lifting to hold up for longer periods. Slowly progress to resting your hands on chest and clasping hands behind the head.

Abdominal massage: is very essential to avoid lines and wrinkles during the third trimester of pregnancy. Start massage from lower abdomen making slow, gentle, circular strokes with both hands over the bulge. This is particularly comforting towards the end of pregnancy. Start again at the sides, using the same strokes and continue up to under the breast fold.

Buttocks

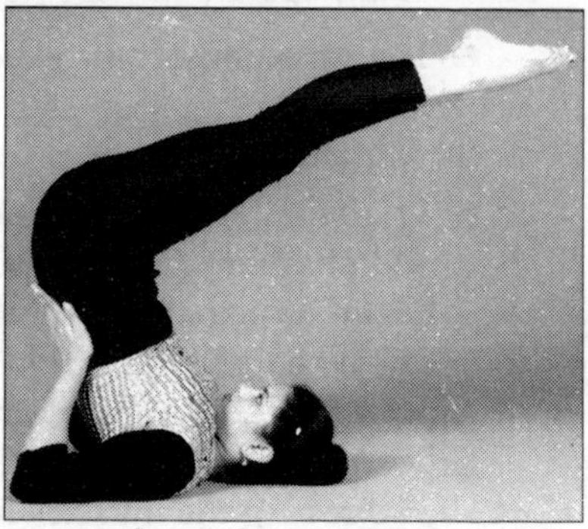

The buttocks play an essential part in supporting the trunk and the growing weight of the baby as, together with the abdominal muscles, they control the tilt of your pelvis. As the abdominal muscles become stretched because of the growing bulge in front, you have to depend more on buttocks to keep correct posture and prevent low back pain. Strong buttocks may also help to prevent sciatica. If they are flabby and collect a lot of fat, or if they protrude at the sides of your thighs, you can take it that they need strengthening of muscles. The simplest exercise is to squeeze your buttocks together slowly for sometime.

Here is another a bit tough exercise for the buttocks:

Lie on your back with your legs bent, feet hip-width apart. Do a pelvic tilt and continue pushing your hips up until your back is in straight line from shoulders to knees. Hold the position for few moments, squeezing your buttocks tightly together. Hold for few seconds, and lower the hips. Repeat three times, twice a day. You can also do this exercise when you are resting on the floor with your legs on a low sofa or bed, keeping the legs straight.

How to massage buttocks?: Tension exists at the lower back and the buttocks. Buttock muscles can be rid of tension with powerful massage movements as below:

- **Step 1:** Work flowing and rhythmic strokes in circles clockwise on right buttocks and anticlockwise on the left buttock gliding hands downwards.
- **Step 2:** Place hands on the buttocks and stroke smoothly up keeping both hands relaxed, twisting inwards from the sides of the waist.
- **Step 3:** Now push hands upward, kneading fleshy buttocks in hands.
- **Step 4:** Apply circular pressures with both hands at the bony base at the spine above buttocks.

How to Fight Wrinkles?

Conventional medicine has lots of ways to fix a wrinkled face. Collagen injections are administered to fill small wrinkles. Laser surgery helps to resurface lined areas. Home remedies are also helpful for reducing wrinkles and implanting more youth in the skin.

Applying aroma mask on the skin have a wonderfully rejuvenating effect on ageing skin.

To start massage, first wash and dry your hands. Then rub your hands together rapidly for at least 36 times to bring energy on your palms. Move your hands over your face in an upward motion, covering your entire face, including your eyes. Your hands should touch the skin gently, without pulling. Move each hand in a circle, beginning at the chin and moving up alongside the nose, over the eyes to the forehead, along the hairline, over the ears and back to the chin again. Do this circular motion 36 times. Follow this technique daily as a part of your skin care daily routine. The following home-made mask, which contains essential oils stimulate the production of new skin cells, thus helping to reduce fine lines and wrinkles:

- **Anti-wrinkle mask:** Mix in a bowl 1 teaspoon each facial quality clay and oatmeal or oat flour, ½ tablespoon powdered milk, 2 teaspoons honey, 1 teaspoon avocado or olive oil and sufficient water to make a paste. Add to it two drops of essential oil of neroli, lavender or rose. Apply the paste in an even layer to your clean face, avoiding the eye area. Leave mask for 10 minutes, it begins to dry after 10 minutes. While the mask is on, lie down with your feet slightly elevated and cover the eyes with moist eye pads. Rinse with warm water. Finally splash cool water. Use the mask two to four times a month.
- **Aromatherapy face pack for sagging skin:** The pack tones a sagging skin. Combine one drop each of essential oils of neroli and primrose oil (or borage oil). Put the mixture on a cotton pad and wipe your face with it after cleansing routine. The essential oils help the skin to regenerate. Primrose and borage oils are rich in gamma-linolenic acid—one of the fatty acids involved in collagen production.
- **Misting to reduce fine lines:** The components in our skin have ability to hold moisture decrease with age. Misting the skin by spraying it with a fine mist of water can help moisturize your face and reduce fine lines. Misting helps soften and plump the dried, wrinkled skin, reducing fine lines. The moisturizing element can be plain water mixed with 10 drops of essential oil or rose water. Essential oils such as neroli,

lavender, or rose oils are very beneficial to enhance skin beauty. Be careful not to spray it into your eyes, since essential oils irritate them. Misting is good for wrinkled, ageing skins.

- **Massage eases forehead lines:** You can reduce the lines on your forehead with a gentle massage. To a base of few drops of sesame or almond oil, add two drops each of sandalwood and geranium essential oils and one drop each of lemon and cardamom oils. Gently massage your forehead using horizontal strokes for three to four minutes once a day.
- **Massage reduces crow's feet:** To prevent and eliminate crow's feet, apply small amount of moisturizer or massage oil to the area around your eyes to enable your fingers to slide without pulling the skin. Use middle finger of each hand for massaging at the inner part of your eyebrows, using slight pressure as you glide over the eyebrow towards your temples and underneath the eyes along the bones. Circle the eyes 30 times. Use this massage once a day.

How to Erase Wrinkles as You age?

The following steps help to prevent or reduce wrinkles:

- Avoid overexposure to sunlight.
- Don't smoke, since smoking deprives your skin of oxygen and nutrients.
- Choose cleansing lotions instead of soap, since soap foams up and make your skin feel squeaky clean strips your skin of natural oils and ages it prematurely
- Limit coffee and alcohol to one cup a day, since more than that can rob your body of water and nutrients, which in turn can age and wrinkle.

Massage therapy to control ageing: Massage therapy is a technique in which muscles and other soft tissues are pressed, rubbed and manipulated. There are several forms of massage. The more common Swedish massage is a gentle form of muscular manipulation used for relaxation and stress relief. Clinical massage therapy treats specific health problems. Pain causes the nervous system to stimulate muscles to contract. The contractions cause more pain, which result in more contractions. Massage is a way of breaking this cycle of pain and contractions. It persuades muscles to relax and lengthen, and brings pain-relieving oxygen and the blood to the muscles, which removes irritating waste materials (toxins).

Massage therapy is effective to all types of body pains in the back, neck, shoulders, legs, thighs, head and other parts on the body caused by tense muscles. Since massage therapy involves manipulating parts of the body, there is possibility that it will make things worse. It is suggested to consult a doctor before turning to massage. Remember, massage should never be done on the areas where there is extensive bruising or any type of tissue damage. You must consult a doctor in case:

- You are pregnant.
- You have circulatory problems.
- You have unusual condition.

Effect of hydrotherapy to control ageing: Hydrotherapy is a technique in which water is applied to the body in order to stimulate and redirect the flow of blood and lymph (the filtered portion of blood that carries waste products away from the cells). Hydrotherapy helps nourish cells and promote the regeneration of tissues, which allow the body to heal from illness or physical damage. Water helps to transport heat and cold. The application of hot water causes arteries and veins to expand and bring additional blood and lymph to an area. The application of cold water makes arteries and veins constrict and push blood and lymph away. These movements of blood and lymph bring in fresh oxygen and nutrients and remove toxins and waste products from the body.

There are many techniques for using hydrotherapy, which may involve use of showers, baths, water-soaked towels and other methods. Daily shower with alternate hot and cold water along the spine helps stimulate the nervous system and trigger improved circulation to the abdomen, lungs and heart. Hydrotherapy cures many diseases, inflammations, infections and obesity. Those suffering from diabetes should avoid hydrotherapy treatment. Always end a hydrotherapy session when you are feeling warm.

Magnet therapy to control ageing: Each cell in a human body has an electrical charge that produces a magnetic field and achieves a healing effect on the skin. A device that emits an electromagnetic field is called as magnet therapy. Applying a magnet therapy can relieve pain, reduce inflammation, heals bones and injured soft tissues including muscles, ligaments and tendons. They are widely used for back, neck and shoulder pain, arthritis, headache, post surgical pain, fibromyalgia, sprains, fractures and other muscle and bone injuries and diabetic neuropathy problems such as insomnia, depression, drug addiction, anxiety, high blood pressure, osteoporosis, glaucoma and neurological disorders such as Parkinson's disease, Alzheimer's disease and epilepsy. Although, magnet therapy is harmless, but the treatment is not advised in following cases without consulting with a doctor:

- You are pregnant.
- You have an pacemaker.
- You have implanted a electrical device.

Effect of yoga therapy to control ageing: Yoga is an ancient and comprehensive form of spiritual self-discovery, which helps to purify and vitalize the body and mind. Yoga therapy is the art and science of healing. Yoga therapy aims to calm the nervous system, which optimally helps to balance the body, mind and emotions. Regular practice of yoga helps to control premature ageing.

Yoga therapy can be very effective in treating all types of muscle and skeletal problems, such as neck and shoulder pain and various lower-back disorders. Practice of yoga asana treats fibromyalgia, arthritis, high blood pressure, insomnia, diabetes, asthma, digestive problems and many of the common complaints of ageing and obesity, besides all major health problems related to stress and tension.

Aromatherapy, Herbal Treatments and Your Age

Aromatherapy is the use of aromas for physical, mental and emotional healing, which severely affect ageing. The primary sources of healing aromas are essential oils distilled from herbs and flowers. Essential oils are volatile, which means that their molecules quickly evaporate into the environment. When you inhale essential oil molecules, they react the brain. Brain plays a crucial role in regulating your emotions, mind and body. When essential oils are applied to the skin, they are absorbed into your bloodstream.

Aromatherapy is particularly useful for digestive complaints, skin problems, infections, stress and emotional upset, hormone imbalances particularly in menopausal women and respiratory complaints (except asthma). Essential oils are extremely potent—much more than dried herbs and should not be applied on the skin undiluted. Pregnant women should not use essential oils during the first trimester of pregnancy, since many oils contain chemicals that may cause an abortion.

Herbal therapy—one of the oldest forms of healings, is the use of medicinal plants for health and healing. Plants contain variety of chemicals beneficial to health. Medicinal herbs can be taken in many forms, extracted and are used in the shape of drinks, foods, creams, compresses, poultices, tablets, capsules and essential oils. Herbal therapy is often recommended for treating chronic conditions, diseases (including cardiovascular, diabetes, arthritis, asthma and many more), illness, healing skin, muscle and other problems.

Self-health Care at a Glance to Avoid Ageing

Nature of disorder	Sign, symptoms and treatment
Alzheimer's disease	A breakdown of brain cells that lead to severe memory loss, confused thinking and personality changes. It gets worse over the time and is always fatal. Patients suffering from this disease can live ten years or more after symptoms first appear. The cause of this disease is still unknown and is more likely in persons over the age of 60. Sometimes, it runs in families.

Common signs and symptoms are the following:

- Memory problems that disrupt normal life.
- Confusion, faulty judgement and reasoning.
- Depression, suspicion and anxiety.
- Neglect of personal hygiene.
- Failure to recognize places and people.
- Finally total loss of memory, speech and physical ability.

Alcohol abuse

Alcohol causes health problems. Excessive drinking can disrupt a person's work, family and social life, and can damage organs in every system of the body—the kidneys, liver, brain, heart and digestive organs. It may increase the risk of many forms of cancer as well. Drinking during pregnancy may cause severe damage to the growing fetus.

Alcoholism is a physical addiction, marked by loss of control. The alcoholic keeps drinking even when it causes physical, psychological or social harm. Here are few signs and symptoms of alcoholism:

- Failure to fulfill work.
- Craving alcohol.
- Loss of control over drinking.
- Broken capillaries, flushed face.
- Yellowish skin.

- Blackouts or memory loss.
- Personality changes including depression, bad tamper, irritability and aggression.
- Withdrawal—headaches, anxiety, insomnia, sweating, shakiness when stop drinking. To prevent drinking, the following steps are advised:
  - Don't drink to try to escape anxiety and depression.
  - Avoid places and events that you associate with alcohol, and don't spend time with friends when they are drinking.
  - Replace your need for alcohol with other activities.
  - Exercise regularly, which can provide sense of well-being.
  - Eat well. Alcohol robs your body of nutrients.
  - Ask your doctor about prescription that may reduce your desire for alcohol.

Anxiety & phobias

Anxiety and phobias are the biggest enemy of ageing. The following are generalized anxiety disorders:

- Severe worry, tension, bad tamper or depression.
- Inability to relax, sleep or concentrate.
- Fatigue and frequent headache.
- Sweating or hot flashes.
- Trembling or twisting.

Signs and symptoms of phobias are following:

- Constant, irrational fear of certain things such as height, blood insects, flying or snakes, upset stomach and general pains.
- Panic disorders such as feelings of terror, racing or pounding heart, chest pain, shortness of breath, dizziness, weakness, sweating, flushes, chills, feelings of unreality or a sense of losing control and fear of dying.

Remedial measures

Treatment can involve drugs, psychotherapy, stress reduction, biofeedback or hypnosis or a mix of these.

- If you are troubled by anxiety, call your doctor.
- Talk to a friend about your fears and feelings. Telling others can release stress.
- Get some daily exercise, such as taking a brisk walk or playing sports or a game. A survey reveals that people involved in regular exercise feel less anxious than those who don't.
- Cut down on alcohol and caffeine. Too much use of caffeine or drugs trigger panic attacks.
- Spend less time in stressful projects.

- Simplify your life by making your schedule less hectic.
- Get enough rest.
- If along with being anxious, you have lost weight and your eyes seem to bulge, you may have thyroid problem or other ailment.
- Learn yoga and meditation. Deep breathing and relaxation exercises may help especially when your anxious level starts to rise.
- Acupuncture therapy triggers the release of brain chemicals that may reduce anxiety and depression.

Arthritis

The primary symptoms of arthritis are pain, stiffness, swelling in and around the joints. If you have these symptoms, you are probably suffering from arthritis. Painkillers used for the relief of pain are very harmful although they give temporary relief. There are many natural treatments that can help to control arthritis pain. Here are few professional steps recommended for the professional care and relief:

- Controlling stress through relaxation techniques and lifestyle changes.
- A complete program of diet and nutritional supplements designed to alleviate arthritis pain and also reduce weight.

- Detecting and eliminating food allergies that may be causing or complicating the disease.
- Creating fungal, bacterial and viral microorganism, including fungal candida that complicates the disease.
- Removes toxins from the body.

The following treatments are recommended to treat arthritis:

- **'Mahanarayanan' oil:** The massage with this oil gives immediate relief. It penetrates the skin and softens pain-causing deposits in the bone.
- The herb 'guggul' can relieve the pain of arthritis within a day or so. Take ¼ teaspoon of 'guggul' tincture with ½ teaspoon of water 30 minutes before meals three times a day. The herb travels to the arthritis bone and removes the imbalances causing stiffness, swelling and inflammation.
- Fish oil capsules available at drug stores reduce the pain. Take 6 gm (or six 1000mg capsules) a day for 4 to 6 months.
- Take one tablespoon of flaxseed oil daily.
- Hydrogenated oils (available in margarine, peanut butter, cooking oils and processed food products) interfere with the metabolism of fatty acid and should be avoided.

- Acupressure provides relief from the arthritis by bringing life energy into the area of the joints. This encourages the flow of blood, which lubricate the joints, carries away toxins, reduce pain, swelling and inflammation.
- Stress increases arthritis pain by tightening muscles. Lie on your back. Bend your knees so that your feet are flat on the floor hip-width apart about 12 inches away from the hips. Keep your shoulders on the floor, but elevate your head slightly with a firm pillow resting your hands comfortably on your ribs and elbows on the sides. Remain in this position for 15 minutes each. This position helps relax the neck muscles and relieves arthritis pain in the spine, shoulders, arms and hands.

Asthma

If you experience shortness of breath, severe coughing spells, wheezing tightness in your chest, excessive yawning or extreme fatigue, you are probably having an attack of asthma. Use your doctor's prescribed inhaler.

Signs and symptoms in case of mild and moderate attack include coughing, feeling of tightness in the chest, noisy breathing and trouble catching the breath. In case of severe attack, the signs and symptoms are rapid, shallow breathing, trouble talking because of rapid breathing and a racing pulse. Monitor your breathing regularly with a peak flow meter, which measures how well air moves in and out of the lungs.

Concentrating on breathing properly can help stop asthma attack. By drawing more air into your lungs, relaxing your body and controlling anxiety and panic you can reduce the severity of attacks. You must sit down as soon as an attack begins. The following remedies are helpful in case of asthma:

- Amino acid n-acetylcysteine (NAC) is a powerful scavenger of free radicals in human body and helps to prevent mucus from accumulating in the lungs. Take 500 mg of NAC twice a day as per recommendations of your doctor.
- Allergies worsen asthma. Quercetin has been scientifically recognized as an anti-allergic and anti-histamine for its properties. Taking 100 mg of quercetin three times a day during six months of allergy season, as per recommendation of your doctor, gives a relief.

Use anti-asthma diets as per detail below:

- Fish contains oil that reduces the airway inflammation of asthma.

- Onions, ginger and garlic strengthen the immune system, which thins mucus.
- Fruits and vegetables are healing components in foods that help control harmful free radical molecules in the body.
- Sea vegetables deliver lot of protein and minerals and leave relieving effect to cure asthma.
- Whole foods supply the best assortments of nutrients, complex sugars, starches and fiber.
- Avoid green tea, which contains substances that dilate the bronchial tubes.
- Magnesium rich foods relax the bronchial tubes.
- Foods high in vitamin C and beta-carotene (especially fruits and leafy vegetables) help fight inflammation of bronchial tubes.
- Track your asthma attacks by keeping a diary. How frequent? How severe? What happened just before an attack? Which of the foods, drugs or actions bring on an attack of asthma?
- When you know that pollution levels are high, keep windows closed and use air conditioner.
- Use a dehumidifier to control humidity. Dust mites and molds trigger allergy. Cockroaches are one of the leading causes of asthma attacks in children. Ward

off cockroaches by storing food in airtight containers.

- U foam leather pillows. Avoid wool blankets.
- Pets like cat or a dog cause asthma attacks. Don't keep pets with hair or fur.
- Do not smoke and stay away from the smoky rooms.
- Exercise regularly, but do not overdo it. If certain exercise triggers asthma attack, try others.
- Lower risk of cold and flu by washing your hands often.
- Practice relaxation methods such as yoga, meditation or deep breathing. Easing stress can reduce the number and strength of attacks.

Burns

Burns leave adverse affect on the skin with symptoms:

- Blisters or burn marks, swelling, headache or stomach pain, trouble breathing, dizziness and loss of consciousness.
- Burns are ranked as first-degree burn (affect only the outer layer of skin), second-degree burns (injure both outer and inner layers of skin), third-degree burn (charred or white skin, which burn down all the layers of skin including nerve endings) and fourth-degree burns, which destroys all the layers of skin to the tissues and organs below. Under such circumstances, take

off clothing or jewellery in the burn area and rush the patient to hospital immediately. If you suspect a heart attack, call the doctor at once.

Cuts, scrapes & wounds Scrapes can hurt, but they usually bleed only a little. Cuts can bleed heavily. Puncture wounds may not bleed much, unless they rupture major blood vessels or organs. Call for the medical advice if a wound is deeper than 1/4th inch, it has jagged edge, if bleeding doesn't stop after five minutes. A cut, scrape or a wound may leave a permanent scar on the skin. Put a cold compress over the wound. In case of minor bleeding, clean the wound with soap and water and cover with a bandage to stop bleeding and to prevent infection.

Chronic fatigue syndrome You probably have chronic fatigue syndrome if you have had fatigue with the following symptoms:

- Short-term memory loss also known as brain fog.
- Sore throats.
- Muscle and joint pain.
- Headaches and un-refreshing sleep.
- Increased thirst.
- Bowel dysfunction.
- Recurrent or persistent infections.
- Tiredness after exertion, which lasts for hours.

Chronic fatigue patients have several health problems including premature ageing. Among these, the prominent disorders are common:

- Disordered sleep also known as fibromyalgia, in which body muscles shorten and become painful.
- Hormone deficiency in the body, which leads to premature ageing.
- Poor immunity that leads to chronic infections including yeast overgrowth, sinusitis and bowel infections.
- Nutritional deficiencies.

Treatment: The treatment involves as sleeping aids, hormone treatments, antifungal and anti-parasitic medication for infections and nutritional treatment.

Dizziness

Dizziness has many causes with the following symptoms:

- After blow to head, neck or back, due to loss of consciousness, headache, nausea and vomiting. See a doctor for treatment.
- In case of fever over 104, rapid pulse, hot, dry skin, the cause may be heatstroke. See a doctor immediately.
- In case of palpitations, shortness of breath or chest pressure or pain, the cause may be a minor heart attack. A complete rest and attention of a doctor is needed.

- In case of sudden dizziness and headache, severe weakness or numbness, blurred vision or trouble speaking due to a stroke, see a doctor immediately.
- In case of a head injury, it causes dizziness, fatigue, weakness or numbness in one side of body. See a doctor immediately.
- In case of a head injury, when there is bleeding and swelling in the brain, see a doctor immediately.
- In case of symptoms such as dizziness accompanied by vomiting, sudden high fever, headache, red rash on the palms of hands and soles of feet due to toxic shock or bacterial infection in blood see a doctor immediately.
- Heat exhaustion while working or exercising in hot weather that shows symptoms such as dizziness accompanied by headache, vomiting, excessive sweating, clammy skin, rapid pulse and cramps in arms, legs or abdomen, call doctor immediately, cool the patient with wet cloths. Give water, juice or re-hydration drink to the patient.
- In case of brain tumour, dizziness accompanied by symptoms such as, frequent headache, nausea and vomiting, double vision, seizures, confusion and memory

loss consult a doctor for examination and treatment.

- In case of hypoglycemia (low blood sugar) with symptoms of dizziness, headache, intense hunger, shaking, irritability, confusion and anxiety, people with diabetes should eat or drink something with sugar in it.
- In case of anemia accompanied by dizziness, weakness and fatigue, and shortness of breadth, see a doctor.
- In case of ear infection accompanied by pain, fever, chills, stuffy nose, muffled hearing, pussy discharge from ears, restlessness and lack of appetite, consult a doctor.

Electric shock

Symptoms include deep, charred or small burns on the mouth or other parts of the body, tingling sensation, sudden dizziness or headache, muscle pains, loss of consciousness or heartbeat. Remove the source of electricity as quickly and safely as possible. Give first aid for the burns. Electric burns are often deeper and more serious than they appear. Cover the patient and make him/her comfortable as much as possible and call a doctor for emergency advice.

Heart attack

Signs and symptoms of a heart attack include crushing or squeezing chest pain or tightness that lasts 5 to 10 minutes and does not ease with rest. It often starts in the centre of the chest, then spreads to jaw, neck, back or arms (more often left arm and shoulder). Women are less likely than men to have severe chest pain. Other symptoms of heart attack are shortness of breath, fear or anxiety, dizziness, sweating, nausea and vomiting, pale or bluish lips, skin or fingernails, uneven heartbeat and unconsciousness. Do not try to move a heart attack patient, loosen clothes, keep the patient warm and seek immediate medical help. If the person is conscious, a sitting or partly sitting posture may make breathing easier.

Hypothermia & frostbite Hypothermia occurs when body temperature falls much lower than the normal. If not treated timely, it can lead to loss of consciousness, cardiac arrest and even death. Usual symptoms are shivering, loss of coordination, clumsiness, weakness, sleepiness or unconsciousness. Long exposure to cold freezes the skin and damage deeper tissues to make you appear aged. Keep patient warm. If the person is conscious, offer sips of a warmed, sweet beverage. Do not give any drink with alcohol. Till the medical help reaches, start rescue breathing, if needed and chest compressions is observed. Loosen tight clothing and remove jewellery. Take following precautions:

- Do not use direct heat.
- Do not massage frostbitten skin.

- Do not smoke or drink alcohol.

Hair loss

Hair loss in men is rarely health threatening, unless it is sudden and occurs in patches over the head. This disease of the hair follicle is called alopecia areata. Usually, men's hair loss is genetic male pattern baldness. Hair loss in women is difficult to diagnose and can be caused by many factors as below:

- Suffering from alopecia areata (patchy baldness).
- Hormonal imbalances.
- Menopause, also known as the change, which usually occur around the age of 50 when the menstruation stops. A menopausal woman experience hot flashes and night sweats, fatigue and insomnia, vaginal dryness and loss of sex drive, depression, memory loss and sudden mood swings.
- Dietary protein and amino acid deficiency.
- Intestinal parasites.
- Damage from the hair treatment.
- Stress.

A woman with hair loss should discuss the proper treatment with a doctor or a naturopathic physician, who usually suggest the following natural treatments:

- When the head is hot, the hair roots become unstable and the hair loss can result. Massage the scalp with sesame oil, which penetrates the skin to lubricate not only the scalp but also the entire body.

- The herb 'gotu kola' is calming and can help slow or stop stress related hair loss.
- Fatty acids found in flaxseed oil, sunflower oil, soy oil, evening primrose oil and black currant oil are effective against the processes that contribute to male pattern baldness.
- A paste made mixing ½ teaspoon of fenugreek powder and ¾ cup of unsweetened coconut milk can energize the scalp and encourage hair growth.
- Aromatherapy works miraculous to stop hair loss. Mix together essential oils in a glass bowl, such as one tablespoon jojoba oil, three drops rosemary oil, three drops lavender oil, one drop of lemon balm (Melissa oil) and one drop of Atlas cedar wood oil. Massage the mixture into your scalp with your fingertips. Leave it on for 30 minutes or overnight, then shampoo in the morning. As a final rinse, add one drop each of rosemary and lavender oil to ¼ liter of cool water and pour it over your head.

Headaches

Frequent headache may result in premature ageing. Sudden severe headache accompanied by paralysis, weakness, numbness on one side of body, nausea and vomiting, loss of consciousness, trouble speaking, dizziness and confusion and fever might be due a stroke. Visit a hospital immediately for a thorough check up.

Headache accompanied by nausea and vomiting, stiff neck, aversion to light and red rash might be due to meningitis. Visit hospital for check up immediately. There might be a brain tumour in case of severe headache on waking or when you lie down with other symptoms such as nausea and vomiting, double vision, dizziness and loss of memory. See a doctor.

In case of glaucoma, the headache is accompanied by intense eye pain, nausea and vomiting and vision problems. In case of sudden, intense headache with symptoms of dry mouth, sticky saliva, fatigue and thirst, this might be due to dehydration or diarrhea. The patient should drink small quantity of liquids often. The symptoms of migraine headache cause severe throbbing pain often on one side of head, vision problems, aversion to light and noise, dizziness, nausea and vomiting.

The symptoms of tension headache include a lasting pain that can be dull or intense, feeling of a tight band around the head, stiffness and tightness in neck and shoulders. In case of symptoms of fever, pain behind forehead and eyes with stuffed-up nose and sinus, there might be a sinus headache. Extreme, non-throbbing pain usually around one eye, bloodshot or watery eye, red face and stuffed-up nose are the symptoms of cluster headache. To treat a cluster headache, apply ice packs and take hot showers. Consult a doctor immediately after initial attacks.

Overweight

Overweight is the symptom of fundamental imbalances in human body, emotions and mind, which include emotional imbalance, nutritional imbalance, physical imbalance and mental imbalance. Reducing weight can help solve various nutritional, metabolic, hormonal, immune and lifestyle problems that cause overweight. There are eight factors as below, which generally cause weight problem:

- Depleted brain chemistry.
- A low-calorie diet, which is common cause of overeating.
- Blood sugar problems, including hypoglycemia, diabetes and exhaustion of adrenal glands.
- Low thyroid function.
- Food allergies and addictions.
- Hormone imbalances.
- Yeast overgrowth and candida, which cause carbohydrate cravings.

- Deficiency of essential fatty acids.

Parkinson's disease

With Parkinson's disease, connections between the brain and muscles become weak resulting in tremors, a stooped and rigid posture, slow and difficult speech, a mask like facial expression and eventually dementia. Conventional medicines, however, slow the progress of disease. There are various nutritional supplements that can help control or delay some of the mental symptoms. Antioxidants come to rescue and slow the progress of this disease and reduce symptoms. Antioxidants can block the free radical damage and slow the progress of disease. Vitamin C starts working first and is replaced by vitamin E and then replaced by glutathione. The recommended daily dose of Vitamin C ranges between 1000 to 1400 mg in three doses. Vitamin E ranges between 600 to 1200 international units a day in three doses. The daily intake of glutathione should be 200 mg. A deficiency of vitamin B12 disturbs mental functioning and 100 microgram a day dose in a B-complex or a high-potency multivitamin/mineral supplements.

Stroke

Stroke occurs when blood flow to the brain is cut off usually because of blocked artery. Timely medical help reduces some of its adverse effects. Common signs and symptoms are the following:

- Abrupt weakness or numbness of the face or body.
- Sudden loss of vision, often in one eye.
- Loss of speech or troubled speech.
- Sudden, severe headache.
- Dizziness, unsteadiness or loss of consciousness.

Seek for immediate medical assistance. Do not let the person eat or drink. If vomit or fluid is draining from the mouth, turn him or her onto the side, so the airway does not become blocked.

8

Slim-trim Figure to Control Ageing

Age Spots

These are brown spots on the body usually due to direct exposure to sun. The ultraviolet radiation damages the colour-producing cells of the skin, which are called melanocytes. In many cases, age spots are cosmetic problems or health threatening conditions. They can be temporarily removed with bleaches, liquid nitrogen or laser surgery. In extremely rare cases, the area of spot can develop a life threatening cancer called melanoma. If one of your age spots or area around a spot has turned black and is irregular in shape, see a doctor immediately. The following natural remedies cure age spot:

- **Aromatherapy:** It helps the spot fade. The essential oils of lemon and benzoin have bleaching properties that can help age spots fade. Combine two to three drops of one of the oils with vegetable carrier oil such as almond, then apply the mixture to the spot twice a day.
- **Natural bleach:** A mixture of honey and yogurt create natural bleach that can help lighten age spots. Add 1 teaspoon of honey to 1 teaspoon of plain yogurt. Apply the mixture to your hands, let it dry, then wash it off after half an hour. Do this once a day.
- **Solution to lighten or eliminate age spots:** Licorice and glycolic acid are beneficial to eradicate age spots.

Glycolic acid contains natural sugar acids derived from citrus, papaya or other foods. It gently exfoliates the top layer of the skin, while licorice bleaches the spots.

- **The herbal cure:** The herb 'gotu kola' may help fight age spots by stimulating the growth of new, healthy cells and production of collagen. Use of tincture or capsule (one or two capsules of 60-milligram) form of herb to ¼ cup of water taken three times a day.

Stretch Marks on Abdomen

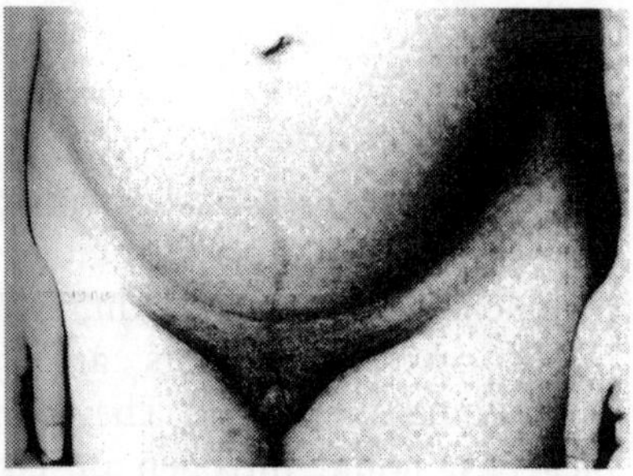

Such marks generally appear after the delivery of first baby. Abdominoplasty is the most modern process to cure these marks. Slim, supple figure is in vogue. Every woman wants to look and feel younger. Lax abdomens, wrinkled faces, sagging breasts, shapeless thighs—all are sources of embarrassment to persons willing to lead an active glamorous life. Aesthetic surgery now offers new avenues to make you look better and younger. If you have lax, shapeless abdomen with extra fat on it, you have a chance to get rid of it by a procedure commonly called abdominoplasty.

Abdomenplasty (body contouring)

It is primarily an aesthetic repair of the abdominal wall and is performed to correct deformities of the skin, fat tissue and muscle. The abdominoplasty technique aims to:

- Permit resection of excess skin.
- Close muscular separation and tighten their laxity.
- Leave a scar that can be sometimes hidden in the groin fold or can be hidden under the bikini suit.

The majority of patients requiring body contouring are females because they are more beauty conscious. Sometime males, too, suffer from it. The main causes are the following:

- Sudden weight loss.
- After the pregnancy, especially delivery of child carried by surgical operation.
- Obesity and previous operations.

The body contouring has become a common process due to the change in lifestyle, mainly due to the following reasons:

- In modern society, emphasis on youth and vigour.
- A more liberal attitude towards sex.
- Fashionable clothes that reveals the body.
- More time spent in leisure and recreational activities.

The following discrepancies have been observed in most of the patients:

- A marred skin.
- Sagging and wrinkled skin.
- The protruding abdomen.
- Social and sexual activities are limited frequently in order to avoid embarrassment of exposure of the abdomen.

Recommended remedial factors to undergo body contouring are the following:

- A vigorous exercise regime helps to increase muscle tone, but it will not improve problem of excess fat on the skin nor will it correct the post-delivery pot-belly.
- The ideal patient for body contouring is a person normal in weight according to his or her stature and height.
- A woman who does not plan further pregnancy.
- A person ready to accept the inevitable surgical scar.

The following precautions are observed when undergoing body contouring:

- Do not take aspirin containing drugs 10 days prior to surgery.
- Discontinue birth control pills and other hormones.

- A careful bath with medicated soap for two days proceeding surgery is advised.
- The choice of surgical technique depends upon the anatomic deformity in individual cases for which consultation of an experienced surgeon is required.

The surgery is conducted in the following ways:

- The skin incision begins just inside the pubic hair line and curves gently to groin skin flap along with the fatty layer is separated from the deeper muscles up to the umbilical level.
- The excess of skin and fatty tissues are excised after locating the umbilicus at the desired level. Post-operative pain and discomfort is usually moderate and limits activities for two to three days.
- The patient is allowed to move after the fifth day. Normal activities are resumed slowly. Vigorous activities like swimming and running are avoided for at least 12 weeks.

Abdominal Massage

Abdominal massage calms the nerves and stimulates the digestive system. If you are suffering from stomach ache caused by tension, indigestion or a bad menstruation, abdominal massage can soothe them. An abdominal massage leaves the following effects:

- Relieves constipation.
- Helps in shedding flab.
- Improves skin texture.

Remember, expectant women are not advised to have a complete abdominal massage. However, a very gentle massage is beneficial for the mother and the child in the womb. Placing a pillow under the knees while massaging helps relax the back and stomach muscles. The following movements are recommended for an abdominal massage:

- **Step 1. (Stroking):** Place your hands side by side on lower abdomen and move them slowly up towards the ribs with even pressure. Mould the hands to the curves of the body around navel and pull hands firmly at the sides of the waist.

- **Step 2. (Circle stroking):** Put left hand on the lower ribs and start massaging with right hand below the navel, stroking gently towards the left hand circling the navel in clockwise direction exerting very smooth and light pressure. Use both hands for the massage. Glide your left hand round the waist while the right hand may be used to stroke up the abdomen in circles, gently and rhythmically.
- **Step 3. (Rotary pressure movement):** Press down with both hands in circles gently. Release the pressure and glide smoothly in the adjoining area around the navel with rhythmic and firm pressure.
- **Step 4. (Kneading):** Start from the hip with both hands facing each other squeezing and releasing the flesh. Work thoroughly over the whole hip with deep and stimulating kneading movement.

Obesity and Cellulitis

Overweight is the symptom of fundamental imbalances in your body, emotions and mind. These imbalances include the following:

- Emotional imbalance.
- Nutritional imbalance.
- Physical imbalance.
- Mental imbalance.

To help you lose weight, a person should understand and in a position to solve the various nutritional, metabolic, hormonal, immune and lifestyle problems that cause overweight. The practitioner should be able to medically investigate and correct the following factors:

- Depleted brain chemistry.
- A low-calorie diet, which is a common cause of overeating.
- Blood sugar problems including hypoglycemia, diabetes and exhaustion of adrenal glands.

- Low thyroid function.
- Food allergies and addictions.
- Hormone imbalances.
- A deficiency of essential fatty acids.
- Carbohydrate cravings.

A holistic approach to overcome overweight

- **Food — that stops cravings:** Have light smoothie or blender drink for the breakfast. You may prepare an important balance-restoring weight loss drink for the breakfast by blending the following ingredients:

Rice milk	1 cup
Soy milk	1 cup
Apple juice, orange juice	1 cup
Banana	1
Strawberries	4
Blackstrap molasses	1 teaspoon
Aloe juice	1 tablespoon
Black cherry juice (concentrate)	1 tablespoon
Powdered green formulation	1 tablespoon
Powdered brewer's yeast	1-2 tablespoon
Raw, organic bee pollen	1 teaspoon
Flaxseed oil	1 tablespoon

- **Take smaller quantity of food:** Continue with balanced diet. It should be quality food, not quantity food. Be sure to include reasonable amounts of potatoes and whole-grain cereals in your diet.
- **Eat slowly:** This helps to digest food quickly.
- **Avoid heavy foods:** Do not eat foods, which are oily and high in fat.
- **Be careful about leftovers:** Many housewives put on weight because they do not like to see food wasted. It is better to cook less food, which is likely to be consumed.

- **Live on reduced diet:** Stop nibbling between meals. There should be three diets in a day and avoid eating in between the meals.
- **Sensible exercise:** Take regular daily exercise, this will help to use up those extra calories. Walking is an excellent exercise to maintain slim body.
- **Avoid rich desserts:** All that excess sugar and fat is high in calories but low in food value. Your best exercise is to push yourself away from the dining table while you are still hungry. Do not eat ice cream, pastry, rich cakes and sweets.
- **Regular eating:** Remember, a regular eating is important. Your meals should be smaller than average, well prepared and attractively arranged on the dining table.
- **Do not go hungry for long:** Eat regularly but sparingly — the best way to lose weight.
- **Be sure to have regular breakfast:** Many people slip their breakfast. Have a good breakfast, this will carry you through the day and you will be less tempted to nibble sweets and snacks between the meals.
- **Recommended foods:** Green leafy vegetables, tomatoes and carrots contain less calories, but are high in vitamins and minerals, and possess real food value.

How to Fight Cellulite?

Cellulite is a combination of fat globules, waste matter and water imprisoned in connective tissue. Cellulite begins on the inside surface of the thighs and knees covering up the bone projections. It quickly moves down to thicken the ankles, which disappear from view. This thickening spreads and soon affects the whole leg from ankle to knee. The thickening spreads to the lower limbs and the sides of the thighs swell out. Then the hips become heavy with the rolls of fat, as do the buttocks. From there it spreads to the rest of the body and produces thick necks, swollen napes, heavy shoulders, the back of arms, shoulder-blades, spinal column, on the forehead and the lower part of the face.

Symptoms of Cellulite

- Pinching the skin painful and produce small wrinkles and bruising.
- Badly nourished appearance of the skin, which looks rough, grayish and cold.
- The skin gives a feeling of padding.
- The skin adheres to the underlying tissues, instead of being loosely separated from them.

Lotions and Potions

Certain herbal formulas have restorative powers that can help smooth skin affected by cellulite. Massage with aromatherapy oils, which are readily available in health food shops, are absorbed directly through your skin and combat cellulite. Following home remedies help to fight cellulite:

- Eat plenty of fresh fruit and vegetables, which are low in calories, yet packed with nutrients. Drink fruit and vegetable juices daily.
- Eat a healthy, balanced diet.
- Relax in your bathtub. Add 2 cups of sea salt to warm bath water, which will leave your skin feeling smooth.
- Combat constipation. Your meals move more quickly through your digestive tract when you eat plenty of high-fiber foods like green vegetables and grains.
- Avoid plenty of late-night snacks.
- Drink beverages at room temperature rather than ice-cold.
- Drink lot of distilled or mineral water (at least 6 to 8 glasses a day).
- Avoid drinking coffee and smoking as far as possible.
- Dry brush your skin, which helps to improve your circulation. Rotate brush gently in circular movements.

- Apply gentle, kneading massage on and around thighs and inside of knees.
- Stay calm as cellulite builds up when muscles get tense and one feels stressed. Try yoga exercises to relax your mind.
- Take a deep breath. The oxygen helps burn fat. A deep breath also helps clean out toxic carbon dioxide from all your cells in the body.

Heavy Breasts

Breasts play a vital part in a good figure. Just as small breasts make a woman diffident about her figure, on the other hand large ones too sometimes lead to a lot of embarrassments. With modern plastic reconstructive techniques, mammaplasty can alter the contour and size of the breasts. There are no muscles in the breast themselves. They consist mainly of mammary glands and fat. The breasts are held in position by the skin and by fibrous tissue, which connect the bosom to the pectoral muscles. Exercises are similar whether you want to increase or decrease the size of the bust. The only difference is that if your bust measurement is too large, you should exercise fairly rapidly. The main causes of heavy breasts are the following:

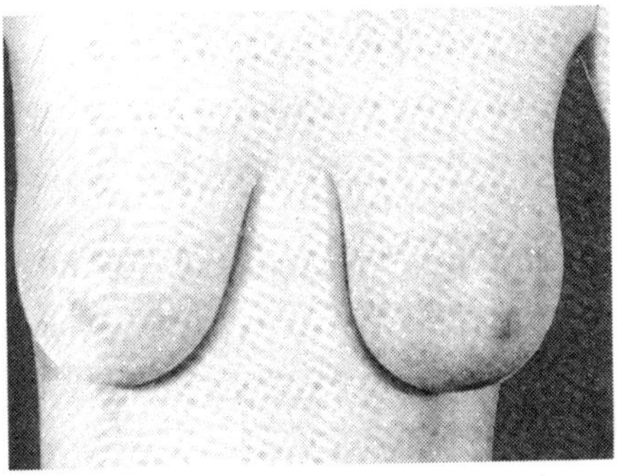

- **Over-development in puberty:** Female hormones cause breasts to grow rapidly during puberty. Sometimes, the breasts may grow to a pathologically abnormal size.
- **Pregnancy over-development:** During the first trimester of pregnancy, the breasts become enlarged and after the delivery, with skin stretching the breasts sag, even though they may regain their former size.

- **Over-development due to obesity:** Usually, women suffering from obesity have over-developed breasts. This is known as 'fatty macromastia'.

The gland fat relationship changes during menopause and fat largely replaces the glands leading to a change in the size and shape of breasts after maternity. Largeness of the breasts depends upon the size of the patient. People with abnormal, enlarged breasts feel the following symptoms:

- The weight of the breasts puts a strain upon the cervical and thoracic spine producing neck pain and backache.
- The brassiere may seem a painful embodiment during the menstrual period.
- Sagging of the breasts also creates problems between the lower part of the breasts and the chest wall.
- Fitting of the clothes needs extensive alterations.
- Breast over enlargement prevents movements and hard work.
- It destroys glamour of the body.
- Due to heavy breast weight, there is always pressure of the bra on the neck or nerve plexus.

What is Mammaplasty?

Mammaplasty is a modern cosmetic surgery, which is too costly. It is a plastic surgical procedure of breast reduction and is performed in case of over-development of breasts by reducing excess breast tissue. Sometimes, this is done in combination with lifting the glands if it sags and the process is called mastropexy. With modern cosmetic surgery, the breast can be reduced to a desired size. With this process the short, narrow scars of the operation are well concealed. The operation is done under anesthesia. With breast reduction techniques, there is no change in the feeding capacity of the breast unless large amount of tissue is excised. Some people fear that the breast reduction will increase their chances of having breast cancer, bur various studies conducted in this regard show no evidence of this.

How to Improve the Bust Line?

In the overall beauty, charm and grace of a woman, no other part of a woman's body is so attractive and enjoys the supreme position, as her breasts. The first thing that attracts an onlooker is the bust line of a passing woman. Shapeless, small, sluggish or over-developed breasts rob the attraction of a streamlined figure. Lifted, well-rounded, shapely and stiff bust of a woman gives her an added attraction and such a bust symbolizes the youthful beauty of a woman. With the passage of youth, the bust gets drooped but if this occurs in youthful days, early attention should be paid to avoid the defects.

Breast care is very important especially for feeding mothers. If a woman's breasts drop and become flabby at an early age, it will fail to give necessary sexual perception. Rightly said by a doctor, what is the use of a breast which is neither useful to the husband, nor to the child. In a natural course, the breasts of a woman should remain stiff and lifted till the age of 50. Ill health, careless feeding of the child are the few reasons responsible for such defects.

To cure mottled looking skin on the breasts, stimulate circulation with alternative rinses of hot and cold water. It will help to minimize the problem and make your bosom firmer. If the skin looks wrinkled and sagging, usually after the childbirth or during breastfeeding, use a good moisturizing cream. In case there is normal delivery, a woman can start taking few light exercises.

When to Start Wearing bra?

At the age of 13 or 14, a girl should start wearing a fit brassiere, which helps to keep the breasts in proper shape. If the breasts are petty or bulky, readymade brassieres of different sizes are readily available in the market and these brassieres help in keeping up the youthful bloom. Always select the brassieres of correct size. Correct size bra helps to keep the breast in place. It should be neither tight, nor loose.

Superfluous Hair on the Breast

This is a common problem in women. With the age, you may even have a very hairy growth between the navel and pubic area. It is unwise to try to remove hair on the breasts and stomach yourself by plucking, shaving or depilatory creams. Electrolysis is the best method and is quite safe for removing permanently unwanted hair from the breast and other areas on the body. Choose a time for the treatment when you won't be wearing a swimsuit for quite sometime. This will give the tiny scabs time to heal properly.

Breast suckling

Some women totally lose the shape of their breasts after the delivery of baby, especially those who breastfeed their child. It is seen breasts start sagging and loose tautness due to the following reasons:

- After childbirth.
- Due to long illness.
- During pregnancy.
- Because of irregular periods.
- During breastfeeding.

Such women are advised to massage their breasts gently daily with olive oil before taking a bath. Breast care is very important especially for feeding mothers. Breasts sag if the infant suckles while sitting or reclining in a faulty posture. For example, suckling with the infant in the lap or suckling lying down is harmful for breasts. Always let the child suckle in a sitting position with the child in the lap and your hand under its head so as to lift it and keep its head steady. Press breast nipples immediately after the suckling and remove the remaining milk with a couple of jerks. This gives lightness and freshness to the breasts. Bathe the breasts with hot and

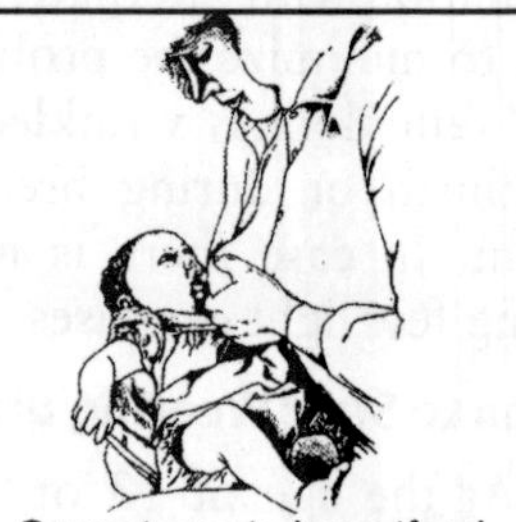

Correct way to breastfeed

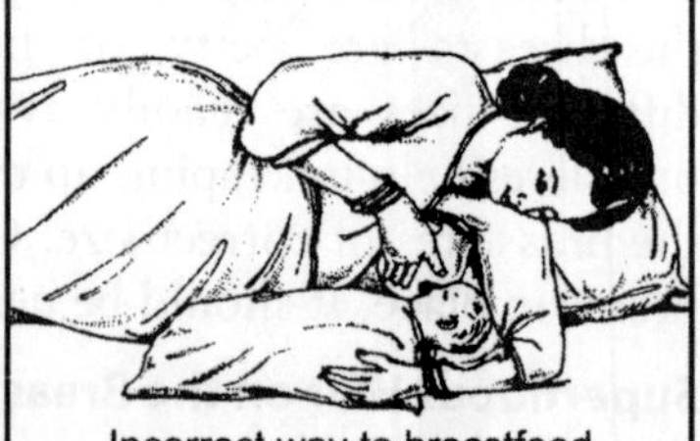

Incorrect way to breastfeed

cold baths simultaneously to ensure rapid blood circulation. Sprinkle hot water and then cold four to five times alternatively.

Wear a well fitting bra while exercising. Some women do not wear any bra at all. Mind, this will further spoil the shape of the bust line. Swimming is an ideal exercise for improving the shape of the bust (especially breast stroke or back stroke). If you can't swim, you can make the arm movements standing in the water. In fact, pushing against water will give the exercise more effect. Always feed the baby on both breasts otherwise a peculiar problem of one breast being smaller than the other develops.

Weight and Height

If you are underweight, the problem is not quite so simple although expert dieticians are almost all united in their belief that if you eat more calories than your body uses, you must put on weight. If you use more calories than you take in, you must lose weight. We all burn up food at varying rates and this is what makes the difference. Some people have an inner boiler that goes on working at a tremendous rate and these are the ones who can eat a plate of cream cakes or a box of chocolates without giving a thought to their figures.

Generally speaking, if you want to put on weight then you should eat all the foods, which those who want to slim must avoid. You can — and should eat wholesome, nourishing meals rich in protein as well as carbohydrates and high in calories. Porridge, cereals, whole-meal bread, butter and jam can all form part of your breakfast in addition to bacon, eggs and fried bread.

At lunch or for the dinner, you should eat potatoes or meat with sauces and gravy. You can start with thick soup if you wish and finish with steamed puddings or custard. Drink plenty of milk all through the day or milky drinks. Aim at several small meals rather than three big ones if you wish to gain weight. Always eat slowly and allow time afterwards for digestion.

In case, you are not gaining weight inspite of all care, you ought to at least have a complete medical examination to be sure there is nothing seriously wrong to their health. Such people should have a complete X-ray of the digestive organs to rule out the possibility of some hidden disease. A stool examination will check the possibility of worms, some amoebic infection and other harmful parasites. A complete blood count is recommended to be sure there is no anemia. The urine should also be carefully checked to eliminate any infection in the kidneys or bladder.

Treatment to Gain Weight

- Multi-vitamin tablets may help to increase the appetite and return body's functions to normal.
- Avoid taking snacks just before meals, for this often spoils the appetite.
- Eat a well-balanced meal, keeping on a high-calorie diet as much as possible.
- Avoid the use of tobacco, particularly just before taking meals.
- Learn to relax. This will help to reduce nervous tension while bringing the body's activities back to normal.
- Have a quiet rest before the evening meal and before lunch. This brings back life and vitality to the whole body besides reducing tension.

How to Grow Taller?

Normal growth is an amazing process. From the moment of conception until the day we are born, growth is extremely rapid in the womb. After birth, a child continues to grow rapidly for the first two to three years, then the process begins to slow down. Once again, around 13th or 14th year teenagers begin growing rapidly. This is the time known as adolescence. Girls grow more rapidly than boys because their hormones are more active in early puberty. Later, the boys catch up and overtake them. They reach their full height between the 16th and 19th years.

A person's height depends to a large extent on the length of the long bones in his or her lower extremities, particularly in the thigh and in the leg. For good stature, the spinal bones or vertebrae must also be well developed in proportion to these long bones. Near the ends of the bones, there is a transverse area known as the epiphysial line, consisting mainly of cartilage in which the bone cells are growing. During childhood and youth, these bone cells are continually adding to the length of the bones. This is how we gain in height and weight. However, growth in height is not steady throughout the childhood and youth. It depends on the changes in the endocrine organs.

Hereditary factors, mental slowness, fatigue and also menstrual disorders (in women) often delay body growth and development. Growth failure in children may be due to several other factors such as child's diet lacking in essential nutrients, inadequate intake of calories, certain diseases involving such organs (liver, kidneys, pancreas, heart or lungs) may all contribute to a failure of normal growth.

Spotty Back and Slim Waistline

Dark complexioned, blemished, unattractive and spotty back is a common problem for women as this is the most neglected part of the body. Usually, men and women take care in beautifying their face with cosmetics and make-up, but a glance at their back proves disappointing as if a beautiful picture is left incomplete. Since the back is exposed because of the styles of the blouse, low back and backless dresses in vogue. It is now essential to take care of back too from the very beginning. The spotty skin, flabbiness due to general obesity and the hair growth on the back are all conditions detrimental to beauty.

The unwanted hairy growth on back can be hidden by bleaching. Spotty backs are often a problem for people who tend to have greasy or combination facial skin. The over-active sebaceous glands that cause the greasy secretions, which starts the spots, are themselves stimulated by hormonal activity in the body, particularly in the adolescence. The following remedial precautions are taken:

- Keep the skin scrupulously clean by washing with a medicated liquid soap daily.
- Change the clothes next to the skin everyday.
- To avoid unnecessary irritation, choose cotton clothes for the vest, bra, blouse or T-shirt.
- Apply a medicated cleansing lotion and an anti-acne cream to dry up the excess grease at bedtime.
- If a spot appears on your back just before you plan to wear a low-backed or backless dress (usually during a fashion show, modeling or a function), disguise it with medicated make-up stick matching your skin tone. It is essential to take care of your back in case you are participating in a modeling session and the back is exposed.

It is agreed that scrubbing and cleaning the back is not so easy, which results in accumulation of layers of dirt on the back but some measures are to be evolved to clean it. Particularly, women with oily skin suffer more as the skin gets black patches and rashes due to dirt. This part becomes itchy and when scratched, irritation increases and rashes spread leaving permanent marks. Those suffering from dandruff in the hair, get it on the back also. It leaves blotches and since the area cannot be reached easily for cleansing, the entire back becomes dark. The following precautions are recommended:

- To give cleaning effect on the back, use a scrubber at the back.
- Medicated soaps are available to heal rashes due to dandruff for cleaning the back.
- Rub in some acne lotion at night.
- Wear loose dress to avoid itching.
- Massage with mustard oil before bath. Wait for 10 minutes and then scrub well.
- Rub back with a paste of 'maida' mixed with milk. Do not use boiled milk, which causes growth of superfluous hair. Leave the paste for 10 minutes, then

dry wash off with warm water. This clears the skin complexion.

- Scrubbing with lemon is also effective for dark back. Cut a lemon in two pieces and rub them on the back. Let the juice dry for 10-15 minutes and wash off with cold water.
- You should do a back facial once a week or once a fortnight. Use of face pack on the back ensures a beautiful, soft and lustrous skin.
- Try gram-flour (besan) pack on the back, which is mixed with rose water and milk. Mix to it a few drops of hydrogen peroxide and mustard oil. Rub the pack on back and other places. Let it dry for a while, then wash off. It has a magic effect to clear the skin.
- Use a hard bed when sleeping to add attraction to your back.
- Keep straight while walking.

Back massage: Back massage leaves a relaxing effect on the muscles of entire body, lowers stress level, relieves backaches, relieves tense and knotted muscles, calms nerves and nervous system with slow, rhythmic strokes and invigorates the nerves with fast, brisk movements.

- Start with stroking movement on the lower back and pressing both sides of the spine with relaxed hands.
- Apply massage by fan stroking (alternate stroking) on the back. This movement, similar to stroking movement improves circulation, warm and soothe the skin.
- Kneading movement is applied with handful of flesh in both hands. Start at the hips and work up the sides of the body on left side followed by the right side.
- Continue kneading movements at the back of the neck, shoulders and upper arms to relieve tensed skin tissues.

- Now relax muscles on either side of the spine with firm pressure exerted by the pad of thumbs. This movement is known as Pressure stroking.

How to Slim Waistline

To slim the waistline practice, any type of bending or stretching exercise you know. Particularly effective exercises, which combine stretching and bending with twisting or swinging around at the waist are useful to make waist slim and trim. You can combine working by standing in one place and sweeping with wide strokes around you. Sweeping the lawn in this way yourself at the house or working at the desk in your office or keeping legs straight and slightly apart and by staying in one place by the centre of the bed and stretching from head to foot of the bed without moving your feet when you sleep help to slim and trim your waist. Here are few easy-to-do exercises, which can be practiced by aged persons, women undergoing pregnancy and after childbirth when they lose the shape of their waistline.

Exercises to Slim Waistline

- Stand with feet apart. Stretch arms up as high as possible with hands touching. Now swing down and turn slightly so that you grasp the back of your right ankle. Straighten up, stretch high and swing down to grasp the back of your left ankle. Repeat three times each side in the beginning and increase to six times in due course.
- Stand tall with feet slightly apart, arms by the sides. Bend over to the right slowly so that your right arm pushes as far down your right leg as fingertips can reach. Straighten up and bend to the left side. Repeat several times you can easily perform.

Massaging waist: Gently stroke the waist with one hand, then both hands one following the other clockwise. Stroke softly on the sides of waist upwards with one hand after the other till both hands reach the navel. Then gently glide hands towards the abdomen and move down the sides to complete the stroke. Repeat this stroke for four to five times. Then cup your hands over the navel for a few seconds until you feel the heat, then lift your hands slowly.

Yoga to Slim Waistline

Dhanur Asana also known as bow posture has several therapeutic advantages especially to strengthen and slim your waistline and tone up abdominal organs. The pancreas get energized by this *asana*, which has good effect on the secretion of hormones of adrenal gland, thyroid, parathyroid, stimulate the endocrine, pituitary and sex glands, excellent for women suffering from irregular and faulty menstruation, leaving a curative and corrective effects on disorders of the joints, spinal cord, lungs, chest, stomach, abdomen, develop digestive power and take off the extra weight and fat forming around the stomach, waist and hips.

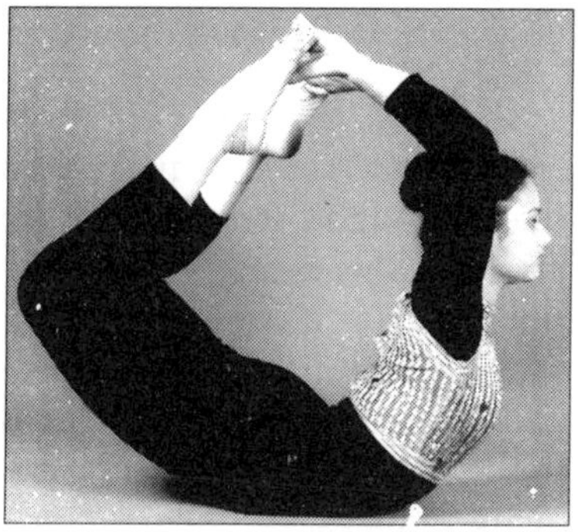

To practice *Dhanur asana*, lie on the stomach with arms stretched on both sides. Place your head resting on left or right cheek. Take ankle in hands, raise legs as well as head and upper part of the body inhaling. Remain in this position as long as possible for you breathing normally. Relax the body and return to the original position. Repeat exercise three to four times.

Trim Your Hips, Thighs and Buttocks

Trim your hips and thighs by rolling exercises, by pummeling them with fists, by standing near a wall and banging hips hard against the wall. This can be done to reduce fatty pads on the thighs. It is also possible to do it by lying flat on the floor or by half lying with the hands on the floor behind you supporting your body. Now raise your hips off the floor and then come downward again on hips. Here is an exercise useful to trim hips and thighs:

Lie flat on the floor, legs outstretched with feet touching arms spread out flat on the floor at shoulder level so that your body forms a cross. Raise right leg until it is at right angles to the body. Then cross it to the left until your right toes are touching your left hand. Keep shoulders flat and still. Return legs to the ground and repeat with other leg. This exercise is very effective to shed off extra fat from your hips and thighs.

Yoga Exercises to Slim Your Hips and Thighs

Utkata Asana is an easy and very effective posture for this. Stand straight, stretch your arms upwards joining palms. Look straight ahead and bend your knees imagining you are sitting on a chair. Have count 5 to 10 times. This exercise strengthens muscles of hips, inner thighs, back, ankles, calves, arms and legs.

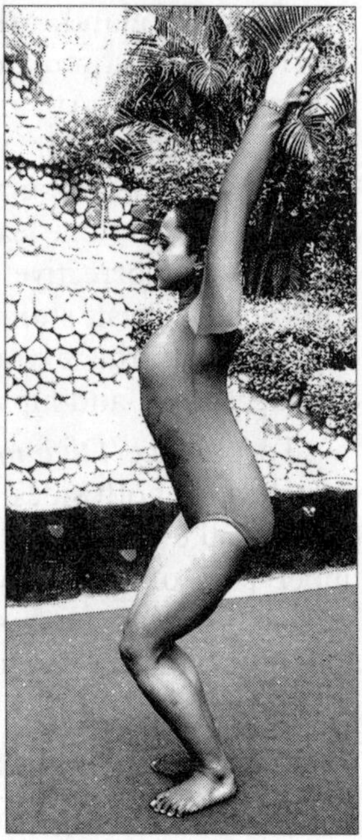

Massaging Hips and Thighs

- Start massaging from ankle to thigh with one hand on each leg moving up to the thighs and hips. Move your hands to the shape of your leg and thigh.
- Knead the thighs rhythmically, squeeze and release the flesh.
- Pummel the thighs and hips with loosely clenched fists of your hands, which bring blood to the surface and relieve stiffness in the nerves. Regular practice of this massage movement is very beneficial to melt extra fat from the hips and thighs.

Massaging the Buttocks

Tension exists at the buttocks. This is usually most neglected area of the body. Buttock muscles can be rid of tension with powerful massage as below:

- **Circle stroking:** Work flowing and rhythmic strokes in circles clockwise on right buttock and anti-clockwise on the left buttock gliding downwards.
- **Fan stroking:** Place the hands on the buttocks and stroke smoothly up towards the direction of back, keeping both hands relaxed. Twisting inwards from the sides of the waist. Now push hands upwards kneading fleshy buttocks in hands. Repeat massage movement several times.
- **Pressure movements:** Apply circular pressures with the thumbs of both hands at the bony base of the spine.

Shaping Tummy

A firm tummy improves the shape of any figure and this means exercising the abdominal muscles so that they will hold you tightly in the same way that a girdle does. One very simple exercise you can do anywhere and at any time simply involves pulling the tummy muscles in and up tightly and then holding them for a count of six. Repeat this exercise after relaxing. If you drive a car, you can do this as a matter of habit every time you stop at traffic lights. You can practice it in your kitchen when you cook and waiting for the kettle or a saucepan to come to the boil. In an office, practice the exercise whilst you are waiting for a telephone call. Any time will do and more often the better. You may practice the following easy-to-do exercises, which are very beneficial for women during pregnancy and after childbirth when the tummy loses the shape.

Exercises for Shaping Your Tummy

- Lie flat on the floor with legs outstretched and feet touching. Place a small cushion or scarf between feet, then slowly raise both legs together until they are at right angle to the body. Then lower both legs slowly. Remember, the legs are raised and lowered very slowly.
- Stand with right hand supported on chair back. Raise left leg until knee is level with thigh. Straighten leg.

Lower the leg after a count of six. Face other direction and repeat with right leg.

Yoga Posture for Strengthening the Tummy Muscles

Ardha Matsyendra Asana also known as *Simplified Yogi Matsyendra Asana* is a simplified version of *Matsyendra Asana*. It is very useful to correct spinal deformities and make tummy slim. This posture has beneficial effect on the gall bladder, spleen, kidneys and bowels. To do this posture, sit straight and stretch both legs in front breathing normally. Fold right leg at the knee by pulling it backwards over the right thigh standing upward and raising the right side buttock.

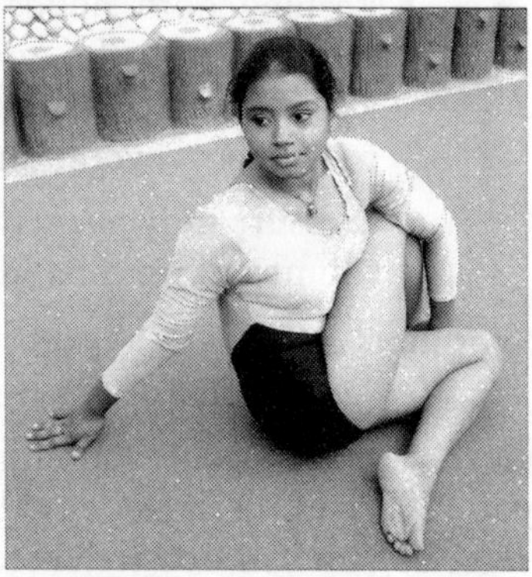

Keep right leg standing and bring the right arm and hand on the back loosely. Now turn the head, chest and waist towards the right side twisting the body as much as possible.

This posture has beneficial effect to strengthen the bones and tone up the muscles of tummy region, abdomen, stomach, intestine, pelvic region, kidneys, spleen, liver, spinal cord and energizes the body.

Hands and Feet

One can guess the age of a person from the skin and shape of hands and feet.

If the skin of your hands is very dry, dull and rough, burn and itch, the following easy home recipes leave a magic result to beautify and protect the skin of your hands:

- Add a few drops of lemon juice and glycerin to a tablespoon of milk cream and rub on your hands at night before going to sleep.
- Massage hands and fingers with almond oil at night before going to bed, which makes the skin attractive.

- For rough hands, take a spoonful of sugar and lemon juice and rub it on the palms till sugar dissolves. Wash off with cold water. Honey can also be used instead of sugar.
- If your skin has been damaged due to ill effects of hot water, soda, washing soap or detergent then wash the hands with vinegar mixing to it water.
- Glycerin mixed with rose water when rubbed on hands with cotton wool swab cleans the skin fantastically.
- The skin is too dry, add carbolic acid to Vaseline (greasy cream) and rub your hands.
- Wash hands with super-fatted soap. Look for the soap that contains emollients.
- Water is the biggest culprit to hands, especially in combination with soap and detergents. Moisturize your hands immediately after washing your hands, which help to prevent drying and chapping.
- Wear protective gloves.

Rough feet can be attended by dipping them in hot water mixed to it a little soda bicarbonate. Scrub the rough parts and heels with pumice stone. Tender parts of the feet like toes should be scrubbed with a nylon brush. Wipe your feet with a clean, dry towel and sprinkle talcum powder on them. Feet have a tendency to sweat profusely particularly if you wear shoes and socks. Sweat dries the skin. Dry skin should be rubbed with cold cream. Sprinkle some deodorant between the toes. Keep the socks clean and wash them after each wear.

Sometimes, there is tiredness, swelling and itching on the feet. For swelling, an effective remedy is to massage them with lemon juice or camphor spirit. In case of itching, wash the feet frequently, dry them and sprinkle powder. If knots are there, apply glycerin on heels and toes, and wash off after 30 minutes. Rub honey on heels before taking bath. Have Foot Bath if the feet are tired.

Foot Bath involves standing in cold water for one to two minutes. In hot Foot Bath, keep feet immersed in a bucket containing hot water at a temperature of 40-45°C for 5 to 15 minutes depending upon the condition. Besides providing relief to tired feet this bath helps to stimulate the muscles of the uterus, intestines, bladder, pelvis and abdominal organs and restores menstruation among women.

In case of cold Foot Bath, immerse feet in cold water having temperature of 7.2 to 12.7°C for one to five minutes. A cold Foot Bath relieves cerebral congestion and uterine hemorrhage and helps in the treatment of sprains, strains and inflamed bunions. Avoid cold Foot Bath in case of inflammatory conditions of genito-urinary organs, liver and kidneys.

Breast Beauty

Fibrocystic: A breast disease in women is common when the breasts are lumpy, cystic or painful particularly around the time of their periods. It is not a disease, but a physiological condition of female hormones during this time of month. There are lot of factors that can aggravate benign breast changes and help keep the pain and lumpiness under control.

- High-fat diets raise estrogen levels in the body and excess estrogen causes the buildup of fluid and cellular tissue in the breast that leads to lumps and pain. Some dairy and poultry products contain hormones that may worsen breast pain and lumps.
- Soy contains natural estrogen, which balances out the excess estrogen in the body helping to decrease breast pain and lumpiness.
- Fiber escorts excess estrogen out of the body. Vegetables such as cabbage, broccoli, kale, brussels, sprouts and turnips help block estrogen from binding to breast tissue.
- Iodine blocks estrogen from sticking to its receptors in the breasts.
- Caffeine in coffee and other sources such as tea, cola, chocolate stretches blood vessels, irritating nerves and increasing breast tenderness.

- Vitamin E helps regulate excess estrogen (Recommended dose include 400 international units twice a day).
- A gentle massage can help improve circulation to the breasts and decrease pain. Make small, gentle, circular motions over the entire surface of the breasts. When you feel a cyst or a lump, massage gently around it. Do not apply hard pressure that irritate the tissue or cause pain.

Engorgement of breasts: The ducts in breasts get blocked causing redness, irritation, tenderness and severe pain. The lactating mother feels difficulty in feeding the baby. Expressing milk is useful to relieve engorgement. The mother should keep up feeding the baby after expressing some milk.

Expressing breast milk: To express breast milk, wash your hands thoroughly. Sit or stand comfortably and hold the container near your breast. Put your thumb on the breast above the nipple and areola and your first fingers on the breast below the nipple and areola opposite the thumb. Support the breast with your other fingers. Now press your thumb and first finger slightly inwards towards the chest wall. You should avoid pressing too far, which can block the milk ducts.

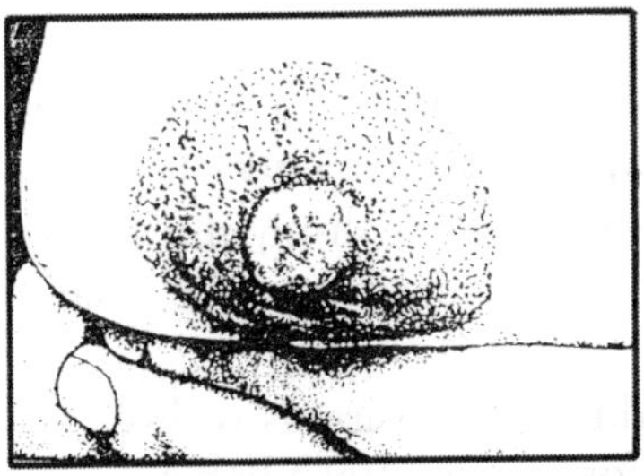

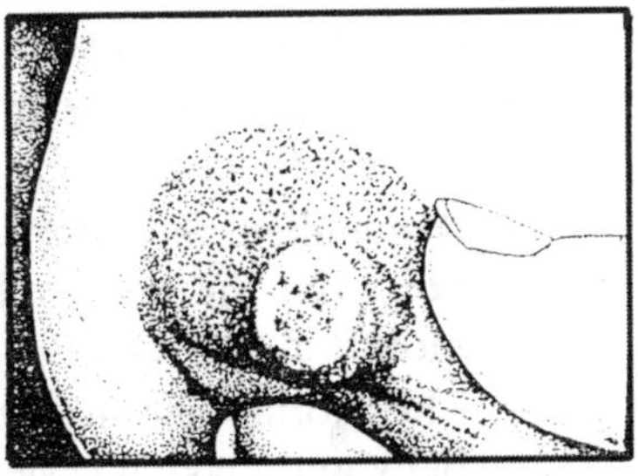

Continue pressing and releasing areola, press and release several times. At first no milk may come, but after pressing few times, milk starts to drip out. It may flow in streams if the oxytocin reflex is active. Press areola in the same way from sides to make sure that the milk is expressed from all segments of the breast. But avoid rubbing or sliding your fingers along the skin. The movement of the fingers should be more like rolling. Avoid squeezing the nipple itself as pressing or pulling the nipple cannot express the milk. Express one breast for at least three to five minutes until the flow of milk is slow. The milk can also be expressed with breast pump. The expression of breast milk is necessary in order to:

- Keep up milk supply.
- Build up constant supply of breast milk.
- Store milk for the baby while the mother is out at work place (in case of working women).
- Relieve engorgement or leakage of milk when the mother is out.
- Keep nipples and skin around the nipple healthy. It is advised that feeding mothers should express few drops of breast milk after a bath or shower and rub on the nipples.

Flat and inverted nipples: This problem is rare after the baby is born. In nearly 4 to 5% cases, mothers are seen to face the problem of having flat or inverted nipples even after delivery of the baby. If the nipple doesn't protrude out, try wearing a shell. Sometimes, the inverted or flat nipples improve and become softer in a week or two after the delivery of child. You may consult a lady doctor also to improve this condition. The following tips are advised:

- The feeding mother should give plenty of skin-to-skin contact to let the baby explore mother's breasts.
- Remember, the baby should suckle from the breast, not from the nipple. The baby needs to take a large mouthful of breasts.
- The mother should try different positions to hold the baby and make it easier for him to attach better.

Mastitis: Severe pain, swelling and block ducts in some area of breast are the main symptoms of a lactating mother. There is often redness, inflammation of breast tissue and tenderness over the lump. If the milk is not removed from engorged breast tissue, there may be severe inflammation — which is called non-infective mastitis. Sometimes, the breast becomes infected with bacteria and is called infective mastitis. The following causes result in mastitis:

- Poor drainage of breast milk after feeding the baby. Express milk completely after feeding the child giving a couple of jerks to the breasts till they are empty.
- Infrequent breastfeeding by the mother.
- Ineffective suckling due to poor attachment of baby.
- Pressure from the bra and tight clothes on breasts.
- Trauma to breasts, which damage tissues and nipple fissures allow bacteria to enter.
- Not lifting the lower part of the breast to help the baby to feed or drain better.

Sore nipples: The main causes of this disorder are the following:

- Improper attachment of the baby.
- Engorgement of breasts.
- Fissures, candida infection, if the skin becomes red, shiny, flaky, itchy, painful and persisting soreness.
- Effect of soap on the nipples or rubbing nipples hard with a towel.
- Applying medicated lotions and ointments on nipples.

To prevent sore and cracked nipples, which can make feeding a baby an unhappy experience, rub the nipples with a mixture of pure lemon juice and olive oil throughout the pregnancy and lactation period. The following tips are necessary for a feeding mother:

- Whilst nursing, add a few drops of essential oil of geranium to a pot of cold cream and soothe the nipples with this.
- Herbs play an important role to prevent sore and cracked nipples. Calendula flowers are useful for clearing the skin of eczema, spots and grease.
- Marshmallow is a herbal remedy for a greater flow of milk.
- To prepare massage oil for the breasts, shake together 4 tablespoons each of apricot and wheat germ oil.

Always massage with warm oil to relieve painful breasts.

- Adding few drops of camphor in 2 tablespoons olive oil makes hard breasts soft when doing massage (while not nursing).
- Mix honey with olive oil or lanolin helps curing cracked nipples.
- Take 1 teaspoon each of dried aniseed (saunf) and marjoram (marwa/sathra), ½ teaspoon each dried fenugreek and honey. Infuse the herbs in 600 ml boiling water for 10 minutes. This treatment improves the flow of breast milk.

Precautions for Breastfeeding Mother

- Keep your breasts and breast nipples clean and dry to prevent them from becoming sore and infected.
- Avoid using soap to clean nipples and areola.
- Do not soak the nipples in water or let them remain moist, this will lead to cracking and infection. Wash the breasts and nipples with water to remove traces of milk sticking to them after feeding.
- Make sure to change the bra very frequently.
- Apply a cream to make breasts and nipples soft (better consult your lady doctor for prescribing a suitable cream).
- Do not apply mustard oil on the nipples to avoid irritation of the skin.
- Before feeding the baby, clean nipples thoroughly.
- Prevent engorgement of the breasts to ensure frequent emptying after a feed. Press your areola so that the milk comes out giving lightness, freshness and correct shape.
- Breasts sag if the infant suckles while sitting or reclining in faulty posture. The best position is to suckle the baby in sitting position with the child in the lap and your hand under the head to lift and keep it steady.

- Bath the breasts with hot and cold water simultaneously. To ensure rapid blood circulation, sprinkle hot water and then cold water for 4 to 5 minutes simultaneously.
- Wear a well-fitting bra while exercising.
- Make sure the areola is in baby's mouth completely and it is pressed when the baby suckles.
- There are wrong conceptions that breastfeeding leads to breast cancer in later life. This is untrue. Rather women who do not breastfeed their babies or remain unmarried have a greater chance of developing breast cancer in later life.
- Nurse from both breasts during each feeding.
- Do not toughen the nipples, which could even do some damage.
- Let your nipple air-dry. Make sure to air-dry the nipples before you cover them.
- If you notice a crack in the nipples, application of vitamin E can help. Take a vitamin E capsule, pierce it, squeeze out a drop and rub into the nipple.
- Try hot compress on the breast to help overproduction of milk. It opens the ducts and the milk flows more freely.
- Control leakage of milk correctly. Press the nipple into the chest. If you leak a lot, find some good reusable 100 per cent cotton breast pads.

Dress Sense Keeps Alive Your Ageing Problem

Dress sense is an innate instinct about what is right and what is wrong. If you don't have this quality, then you can certainly learn some of the know-how by studying fashion magazines, by reading articles on the subject and by watching what fashion-conscious women wear. Don't overdo anything and that goes for the ornaments, accessories and clothes. Keep things in proportion. If you are tall and wearing a heavy coat and hat, don't carry a cocktail size bag. If you are small, keep accessories dainty too and avoid bulky handbag, which will swamp you. Don't have more than two or three exactly matching — for instance hat, bag and shoes or gloves and hat.

Caring of your clothes is all part of being well groomed. This means brushing the clothes at night as soon as you take them off and hanging them in an airy place overnight. Clothes last longer and look new for longer if they are hung properly after wearing and cleaned regularly. Giving clothes time to rest also makes them last longer. Wear clothes in rotation rather than everyday and then changing. Clothes, which are worn rarely should be hung on padded hangers to protect shoulders from marking and they should be covered with polythene bags to protect them from dust. Hang skirts by the loops by using hangers.

Perfume is probably the loveliest accessory any person uses and it can do as much to define her personality and to make her/his remembered as any other part of make-up and dress. In western countries, the liberal use of perfume has always been regarded as an essential part of dressing well and it is very much a part of good grooming. Choice of perfume is important and your own bodily chemistry makes it very personal thing indeed. A fragrance, which smells wonderfully on someone else may be uninteresting or even downright unpleasant on you. No perfume ever smells alike on any two persons.

Choose the type of perfume you wear carefully because the sort of perfume it is can reveal lot about you. Do not spray perfume directly on to your skin, this way perfume can evaporate and the drops are broken up into thousands of microscopic droplets. Transfer your perfume to an atomizer and spray it directly onto your skin, which can't evaporate and settle onto the skin and its warmth activates the skin.

Never choose a perfume by the smell in the bottle. Put a spot on the inside of your wrist, wait a moment for the spirit to evaporate and then sniff gently. If you want to try two scents, put a spot inside the other wrist so that you may be able to compare the merits of both. If you must, try a third by putting a spot inside one elbow or forearm, you will be able to sniff at all three and decide which you like best. Don't try more than three perfumes at a time because your nose will be tired and won't be able to differentiate between them.

Remember that perfume wears off in about the same time as lipstick. So replenish it on your skin, not on your clothes about every four hours. Keep perfume in an airtight bottle in a box or your dressing table drawer as light and air both cause perfume to lose its strength and to evaporate.

Selection of Clothes and Jewellery

A dark complexioned woman should avoid black, blue, pink, light brown and sky blue colors. Instead, orange, red, white and yellow are their well-matched colors. If you like to wear western dresses like maxi, caftan, middy, you should choose printed material. For saris, choose the one with border and 'pallau'.

Although a bride looks beautiful in red dress, the traditional colours do vary as per provincial traditions. Moreover, they can be different in style: sari, salwar-kamiz, lehanga-chunni, etc. Golden decorations on red dress give it a kind of glitter. Make-up is not complete without jewellery. *Beni* on forehead, *zhoomer* or *matha-patti*, *nath* on the nose, earrings, necklace, bangles, *kangans*, *baju-band*, rings, *hath-fool*, *payal* and so on can be worn on this occasion.

For jewellery, go in for diamonds, platinum and silver ornaments, and avoid the ingrained designs. If you are wearing a pallau-border sari, then put on hanging-earrings (jhumka).

Although every type of skin requires proper care, but dark skin needs more care as it requires more moisture than a fair skin. A dark skin develops signs of ageing rather than fair complexion, which is also prone to pimples, shadows, wrinkles and blotches. If you have a dark but dry skin, use a deep cleansing milk followed by a moisturizer at night. Wipe it off with a wet cotton wool swab after 30 minutes. Take a spoonful of un-boiled milk and mix to it little almond oil, a few drops of lemon juice and rose water. Apply the mixture on your face and neck daily at night. This solution is good for clearing the complexion. Use of honey is also good for getting a glow on the skin.

9

Beautiful Body that Affects Ageing

Lines Around the Eyes

The area under the eye is very thin — about 20 micrometer thick. The lower capillaries are not only very thin but have a fine network of blood vessels and tissues. Lack of proper care for this tender part may cause dark circles and shadows under the eyes. They are formed by sluggish blood circulation. This may also account for the puffy eyes.

The skin around the eyes is very fine and delicate and it tends to dry out very quickly. From the age of 25 years onwards, occasionally apply a little eye cream or eye oil to counteract this dryness around the eyes. Do light fingerprinting into the skin above and below the eyes so that you do not see the skin moving if you look into the mirror while you are patting it in. Do not rub your eyes if there is irritation or burning, otherwise the skin will shrink and wrinkles will appear on it. To avoid such wrinkles, use anti-wrinkle cream or almond oil. Here is a home recipe to eradicate lines and wrinkles around eyes.

To remove wrinkles under and around the eyes, start at the bridge of the nose, stroke lightly along the eyebrows with your fingertips, glide towards the temples, then back to under the eyes and the nose. Eye massage relaxes, relieves anxiety and tension. Do not forget to squeeze the eyebrows between your thumbs and forefingers during the eye massage.

Boil leaves of tea in clean water and filter. Soak a cotton swab in it and foment the area around the eyes. Do it every day till you get satisfactory results. Wrinkles and lines are the first to form on the face but they are not caused only by age. They are caused by expression and as such, are known as laughter lines. The upward slanting laughter lines are attractive and give character to the face. The downward sloping angular lines caused by tension, worry and anxiety are less pleasing. With oil or cream slowly massage with your fingers the area around the eyes. Remove surplus cream or oil after about 30 minutes, otherwise your eyes will become puffy. Lack of sleep results in dark rings below the eyes and sometimes the skin becomes flabby. An eight hours rest in a day keep the eyes healthy.

How to do Under-eye Massage?

To dissolve lines and wrinkles under the eyes, following massage movements should be tried:

- Stroke gently with middle finger in a circle round your eyes.
- Work from the bridge of your nose out over your eyebrows, pressing the temples.
- Pinch along your eyebrows from the center to the temples.
- With your thumbs and index fingers, press the bone under the eyebrows at the bridge of the nose.

Pouches and Dark Shadow Under the Eyes

There are several factors behind formation of dark circles or dark shadows under the eyes as below:

- The salt in tear reacts with the skin making it dark under the eyes.
- Lack of sufficient intake of fluids results into accumulations of toxins in the body, which are not flushed out. These toxins leave a harmful effect also on the skin.
- Prolonged illness and long duration of treatment with strong antibiotics cause dark shadows under the eyes.

- Tiredness and improper sleep results dark shadows under the eyes. A man or a woman requires about eight hours sleep every night. Lack of sleep or rest causes tension in the capillaries. The result is dark circles around the eyes.
- **Unbalanced diet:** Regular intake of fatty foods, alcohol and tea or coffee results in total disturbance in the acidic and alkaline balance of the skin. If a person is under-nourished or malnourished, it shows up on the skin in the form of dark circles. Lack of proper vitamins and minerals in the diet also cause dark shadows around the eyes.
- Sluggish blood circulation in the veins of the 'L' capillaries and 'V' capillaries around the eyes, for whatever reason, causes formation of dark circles.
- Damage to the capillaries due to neglect and carelessness results into stressed eyes.
- Disturbed metabolic activities play an important role on eyes. Metabolism plays a major role in having a perfect skin. Metabolic disorders can cause dry/oily skin, dark patches or even dark circles under the eyes.
- Any form of stress or strain on the mind results into improper sleep or rest, lack of appetite, restlessness and tiredness. These in turn strain the capillaries resulting in dark shadows around the eyes.
- Since there are so many different factors causing under-eye dark shadows one must establish the right cause first, to find the correct treatment. To eradicate the problem from the root, it is necessary to deal with it externally and internally, both.
- Sometimes, the eyelids get swollen because of insect bites or infection. To cure it, add one tablespoon of Epsom salt and equal amount of ordinary salt in ½ liter boiled water. Warm this solution before applying it to the eyelids. Dip cotton pad in the solution and apply directly to the swollen lid keeping

it for few minutes, Repeat the treatment for four to five times a day.

Pouches and dark shadows under the eyes make your appearance older by several years.

The skin around the eyes is the most sensitive because the hypodermis, which exists everywhere else, is lacking here. Massage the area gently with fingertips. Never rub your eyes. Instead of rubbing them, blink your eyelids, which gives them the most natural massage. Dark circles under the eyes can be aggravated by fatigue, allergies, overexposure to sun, menstruation or pregnancy. Sometimes, they are hereditary if the parents have them. Sometimes, it is not really darkened skin but engorged blood vessels under the eyes because the skin under the eyes is thinner than skin anywhere else on your body. Usually, dark circles are caused by hyper-pigmentation, higher than the average amounts of melanin — the substance that gives your skin its pigment. The blood vessels there are more noticeable especially when the skin is fair. Exercises of eyes relieve pouches and dark shadows under the eyes. Some of easy-to-do eye exercises are described below:

- Shut your eyes as tightly as you can, then open them as wide as you can. Repeat this exercise 4 to 5 times making sure to keep your eyebrows well lifted. Only the eyelids must move. Keep your forehead and face muscles still. This is an excellent exercise for muscles around the eyes.
- Let the eyes have plenty of rest since night rest is not adequate during the day. Put the palms of your hands over your eyes and relax.
- To keep your eyes sparkling, give them plenty of exercise. Roll eyes around 20 times to the left and 20 times to the right. Take care to close the eyelids when changing direction.
- Another exercise is to quickly blink 10 times. Shut your eyes, keep them closed for a moment. Open eyes and blink. Rest, blink and then rest. Repeat for

10 times. This is an excellent exercise for lubricating the eyeballs and toning up the muscles of the eyelids.

- Look at yourself in a mirror, staring straight at the pupils of each eyes. This is a splendid exercise.

To decongest your eyes, there is nothing like an eye-lotion, readily available in chemist shops. You can seek advice of a doctor in selecting a suitable one. Bathe your eyes keeping them wide open. The lotion moistens the mucus, which is temporarily dried up by the constant action of clearing the eyes of thousands of dust particles.

Remember, dark circles are harmless, but women want to blot them and here are a few easy-to-do tips to relieve them:

- Try a cold compress. Close your eyes and cover them with a cold washcloth for about five minutes. Repeat several times during the day. This will help constrict your blood vessels, minimize darkness and also may help minimize tissue swelling and eliminate some of the darkness.
- Use a sunscreen especially made for the face with a sun protection factor to keep sun's rays away and darken the skin under your eyes.
- Supplement your foundation while doing make-up. For full protection, you will still need a moisturizer or a sunscreen lotion.
- Try eye cream. Alpha hydroxy acids used in many eye creams decrease wrinkles, lighten and smooth the skin. The most common alpha hydroxy acids are glycolic acid extracts derived from fruits and other plants

Puffy Eyes

Puffy eyes may be the sign of something wrong with your general health but if your doctor says there is nothing wrong then check whether you are using too rich and nourishing cream for your eyes and leaving it on for whole night. Creams are beneficial in fingerprinting in this area, but they should be gently wiped off after 15-20 minutes. Crying and lack of sleep are the most common cause for puffy eyes. Sleeping on your face is probably the easiest way to get rid of puffy eyes. You are also more likely to wake up with puffy sacks if you are menstruating or pregnant and retain fluid. Similarly, you may suffer from puffy eyes in the morning if you eat salty foods or drink anything, even water less than two hours before you go to bed. The early morning puffiness can be fairly reduced by alternate hot and cool water bath, and gently patting the eyes and lightly smoothing in a little moisture lotion. Avoid massaging around the eyes until the condition has cleared up. To add sparkle to the eyes and erase puffiness before you start your day, try the following treatments:

- Put 10 chamomile flowers (babuna tree having daisy-like flowers with feathery gray-green leaves) into ½ liter boiling water. They heal ulcers, expel worms, dissolve tumors, banish tiredness and treat many female disorders. When the liquid gets cool, dab your eyes with this solution using a wet pad of absorbent cotton.
- Lie on your back and keep slices of peeled cucumber on the eyes for 5 to 10 minutes.
- Do not rub your eyes. Your eyes will get irritated, red and stay puffy.
- Employ a cold compress. Dunk a washcloth in cool water or wrap ice cubes in a washcloth and place it on your closed eyes. It will help drain the puffs under your eyes.
- Apply a cold tea bag wrapped in tissue on your eyes. Tea contains tannin—a natural astringent and helps pull the skin taut and reduce puffiness.
- Raise your head with pillows while sleeping. Two or three pillows will help keep fluids from pooling under your eyes.
- Avoid alcohol, which makes you retain fluids that can collect in the eye area.

Sore Eyes

Occasionally, an eye make-up product may produce an allergy. Before using eye make-up brush (especially eyeliner brush), check that it is clean. Never use saliva as a solvent. If after using certain aids, eyes get sore or start watering, immediately discontinue with it. Use good quality hypo-allergic products, which do not contain perfume. It is the perfume, which is very often responsible for an allergic reaction. If soreness persists, consult a doctor.

In case of an allergic reaction, in which eyes redden and water and skin around the eyes get a burning sensation, take care to use only high quality products bought from reliable stores or a chemist shop. The markets today are flooded with substandard or imitation products. Avoid using them or you will spoil even your natural charm in a bid to heighten it artificially. Discontinue use of an eye make-up, if your face suffers any trouble like irritation, rashes etc. Always take care to wash your hands well to avoid an infection. Do not forget to remove eye make-up during the night. It is best to use a product, which is gentle and especially formulated for eye make-up cleansing. Baby oil can also be used to clean eye make-up.

How to Take Care of Sore Eyes?

The following steps are advised for internal care of your eyes:

- Proper sleep, for at least, 8 hours a day.
- Intake of healthy and well-balanced diet. Increase the intake of Vitamin A and iron.
- Control on tension and mental stress.
- Metabolic activities should not be disturbed.
- Control intake of carbon, sweets and drinks.
- Avoid heavy, strong and prolonged medication.

The following steps are advised for external care of your eyes:

- Wear sunglasses to avoid sun damage.

- Splash clean water every two hours to remove dirt, grime and bacteria.
- Put two drops of rose water in eyes before going to sleep.
- Apply cotton pad dipped in cucumber juice or potato juice over eyes. This is an idle recipe to remove dark circles under the eyes.
- Massage your eye capillaries with white butter applying light pressure to nourish.

The following steps are advised for a professional care to your eyes:

- Remove make-up before going to bed at night.
- Application of serums and special eye creams.
- Indirect steaming to your eyes.
- Application of a special whitening pack or gel.

How to Remove eye Make-up During night?

- To remove eye make-up, first remove false eyelashes.
- Soak a pad of cotton wool in the eye make-up remover.
- Close your eyes and apply this cotton wool gently from the outer corner working towards the nose. Repeat several times and then open your eyes.
- Using a fresh pad of cotton wool, wipe towards the inside under the lower lashes.
- It is very important to remove every trace of eye make-up before you go to sleep, otherwise it may cause irritation.

Dry Eyes

The causes of dry eyes vary due to overheated room, air conditioned room, air condition car, pollution, working at a computer for hours, grit in eye, allergy due to medicines and above all, ageing factor. More women than men experience dry eyes because of hormonal changes, drop in estrogen production, effect of menstruation and because of menopause. Most women above the age 40 have dry eyes. Every time you blink, your eyes create tears and keep eyes moist and dewy. Dry eyes look red and they burn, tear excessively or feel irritated and scratchy, making the appearance aged. Here are few tips in case of dry eyes:

- Closing eyes for a while doesn't lubricate them. Splash water in your eyes. If you wear contact lenses, skip this remedy, which may lead to infection.
- Apply a cold compress to your eyes.
- Moisten your eyes before blow-drying your hair.
- Drinking alcohol dry out your eyes. Have alcohol to a minimum.
- Smoking is harmful for eyes.
- Wear lenses for a short possible time to ease the strain of dry eyes. Remove you eye lenses at the end of workday.
- If you have scratchy, burning eyes, use tear ointment before you go to bed.

Bags Under the Eyes

If you wake up with bags under the eyes or one eyelid has swollen to three times the size of the other, consult your doctor. It may also be a sign of hives or an allergic reaction due to an insect bite. Also see a doctor if your lids do not close all the way over your eyeballs. It is a possible sign of thyroid disease. Bags under the eyes develop over the years as fat accumulates in the eye area. Unfortunately, once bags form under the eyes, there is no remedy to reduce them. A concealer is more opaque than a foundation to be used. For best results, select a concealer that's just one tone lighter than your foundation.

Akshi Tarpan to Cure Ailments of Eyes

Akshi Tarpan is an important form to cure ailments of the eyes externally.

Long and overexposure to television and pollution along with faulty dietary habits cause several eye disorders such as burning and sensation of the eyes, decreased vision, blurred vision, watering and itching of the eyes.

Akshi means eyes and *tarpan* means nourishment. Therefore, *Akshi Tarpan* is a therapy to provide nourishment to the eyes, which relieves tension in the eye socket, makes eyes lustrous, clears dark circles under the eyes and relieves pain, fatigue, glaucoma, night blindness, inflammation and conjunctivitis.

The therapy involves washing of eyes with medicated *ghee* or oil. For *Akashi Tarpan*, a circular wall is build to surround the eyes. Medicated ghee or oil is poured in the wall up to the eyelashes. *Ghee* or oil is allowed to remain for 15 to 30 minutes depending upon the nature of disorder. *Tarpan* should not be used on cloudy, too hot or very cold days. Persons who are anxious or fearful and have emotional disorders should not use tarpan. If *Akshi tarpan* is overdone, it can cause itching and other *Kapha* disorders.

Correct Eye Make-up

Eye make-up done correctly makes you look younger. The material required for an eye make-up is an eyebrow pencil, eyeliner, eye shadow and mascara. In an eye make-up a sequence followed is — eye shadow, eyeliner and mascara.

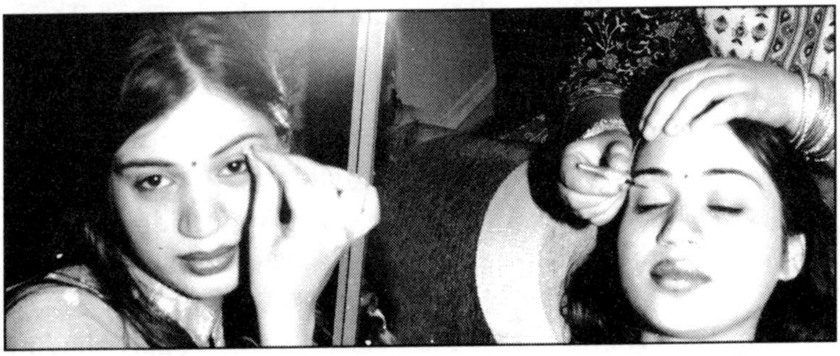

- Eyebrow pencil is used to darken and give shape to the eyebrows.
- Eyeliner is a liquid used on the eyelashes in a thin line. For small eyes, draw a thick line.

- Eye shadow is used on the eyelids between eyebrows and eyelashes applied with fingers. It is also available in many forms like cream, powder, cake and stick. Use a little face powder on the eyelid as a base before using the eye shadow.

How to apply Eye Make-up?

First apply eye shadow on light strokes. Then apply shadow on creases and finally apply shadow on the brow-bone:

Few suggestions for applying eye shadow correctly to beat ageing:

- Most of the Indian women have dark black eyes, and should use chocolate, green or mauve shades.
- During daytime, use eye make-up in light touches.
- Sunken eyes look more sunken with eye shadow, so such women should avoid using eye shadow.
- For protruding eyes, a brownish tinge filled in up to the eyebrows is suitable.
- The eye shadow can make the eyes appear larger or smaller. The round eyes can be made to appear large by extending the shadow beyond the outer corner of the eyes. The small eyes can be made to appear larger by extending the shadow slightly above, beyond and below the eyes.
- For eyes that are set too far apart, use the shadow on the upper inner side of the eyelid.
- For deep sunken eyes, use very little shadow on lids near the temples. Do not apply eye shadow next to the nose and inner corner of the eyes.
- The eyes that are set too close together, apply shadow lightly from the outer edge of eyes.
- The bulging eyes can be minimized by blending shadow over the upper lid lightly up to the line of the brows.

- For heavy-lidded eyes, apply shadow evenly and lightly across the lid from the edge of the eyelash line to the small crease in the eye socket.

Correct Way to Apply Mascara

Mascara is used to thicken the eyelashes. It is available in liquid, cake and cream forms and in large variety of shades used to darken the eyebrows. Apply mascara very carefully in upward strokes on the top of the lashes and downward strokes on the bottom ones applied in two coats. Mascara should be used for an evening make-up with a brush at the root of the eyelashes up to the end.

Take care to clean this make-up at night before going to bed. It is best cleaned with the baby oil. Close your eyes, apply baby oil on a cotton wool swab and scrub slowly and gently from the outer corner working towards the nose. Baby oil is fine if used very sparingly and so long as care is taken, not to allow the oil to trickle into the corners of the eyes.

In fact, application of an eye make-up varies from face to face. You may consult a beauty therapist for proper eye make-up. Use only high quality products for eye make-up. In case of eyes getting red, watery and causing a burning sensation, you should consult an eye specialist and stop using the existing products. It is very important to remove every trace of the eye make-up before you go to sleep, otherwise it may cause irritation.

Beauty of Lips

Every beauty-conscious woman must be aware of the shade of lipstick to be used best suited to the shape of the face, curves of the lips, complexion, hair colour, age and the clothes. Carelessness can mar the looks and makes you to appear older. Lipstick is considered a morale booster and is essentially helpful in giving self-respect and self-confidence. Now even male has started wearing lipstick. Mind, lipstick is used to beautify lips but if applied shabbily, it looks ugly. The following steps are helpful when applying lipstick:

- Before putting on lipstick, clean lips with a piece of cotton wool swab dipped in cleansing milk.

- Never use soap on the lips, as lips have very soft and delicate skin.

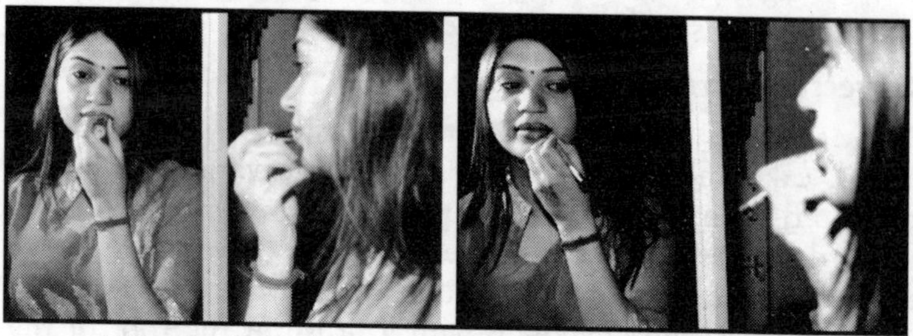

- Apply foundation cream on the lips, let it dry, then apply lipstick
- If lipstick spreads on the lips, apply powder on lips, let it dry and then apply lipstick.
- Use lighter tinge first and then darker for glow. Blend both the colours with a brush.
- Use of Vaseline or cream gives luster to the lips after applying lipstick.

How to Choose a Lipstick Matching Your Face and Body?

Lipstick can change the look of lips. The broad lips can be made to look thin and vice versa and help to mould the shape of lips and your age. The following tips are suggested:

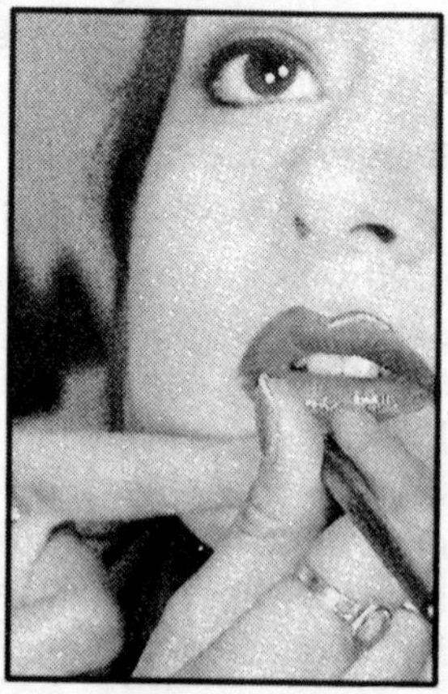

- If you have small face, use light shade on lower lip and dark tinge on upper lip.
- Apply light shade on upper lip, and dark on lower lip, if lips are thin. For broad lips, reduce the outline considerably. On the contrary for making thin lips look broad increase the outline.
- If you have small mouth, draw outer outline with dark shade lipstick and fill in light shade lipstick with a lip liner.
- If you have a broad mouth, use light shade lipstick.

- If your lower lip is protruding out, use dark shade lipstick in the middle of the lips and draw light outline.
- Do not re-touch on a stale lipstick, it doesn't shine or look even, and makes your face to appear aged.
- Remove lipstick before going to bed at night.
- Always use good quality lipstick; sub-standard product can spoil the skin.
- Choose colour of the lipstick as per age, the occasion and clothes you are wearing:
  1. Natural shades suit the teenage girls.
  2. Working women at work place should avoid bright shades as far as possible.
  3. Young women (between the age group 20-25) with fair complexion should use pink shades. Whereas women with dark complexion in this age can use orange shade.
  4. Women between the age group 26 to 40 should choose light shade lipstick.
  5. Colour of eyes is important when selecting a lipstick. For brown-eyed women pink shade lipstick is recommended. If the colour of eyes is black, apply light crimson colour lipstick. For blue eyes, apply scarlet and subdued brown colour lipstick should be used. For grayish eyes, use orange shade.
  6. If the colour of hair is black, use orange shade. In case of gray hair, use pink shade and for golden brown, use scarlet shade.
  7. To choose an appropriate coloured lipstick, colour of the clothes is equally important although it is difficult to match lipstick with each dress you wear. If you are wearing orange shade sari or suit, use pink lipstick and with pink shade clothes, use crimson shade lipstick.

8. You will need a brighter lipstick at night than during the day, because artificial lighting will drain the colour out of the lipstick.

Double Chin

Double chins are caused by excess fat or by combination of excess fat and a loss of muscle tone as you age. Like other facial features, double chins sometimes run in families. Sun-damage, sagging skin further add extra fat to the chin, thus cause double chin. The following steps are suggested to rid of double chin:

- You are not likely to have a double chin unless you are carrying a little extra fat. Try to get back to a healthy weight.
- Eat less and exercise more. Cut intake of calories and increase the amount of physical activity in your life. To cut the amount of food, drink a glass of water before meals.
- Sunrays damage your skin and make problem worse. Apply the sunscreen to your neck as well as on the face every day.
- Follow the neck massage stroking with both hands up the neck from the shoulder to the ear. Repeat five to six times. Now stimulate the jaw line by patting and slapping under the chin, under the jaw line using middle fingers. Finally, soothe the massaged skin with gentle stroking.

Cellulite

Cellulite is fat. You can develop it when you gain weight or when your skin gets a little lax from ageing or lack of exercise. The essential difference between cellulite and fatty obesity or watery obesity is that it affects only certain limited areas on the body, whereas fat and water invade large areas of the body. A woman with cellulite may have it only on the hips or the nape of her neck or in both legs, the rest of the body being unaffected. Cellulite is an inflammation of the connective tissue caused by poisons accumulating there instead of being thrown out by the body. The most common of these poisons are uric and oxalic acids. In case of cellulite, the double chin, thick shoulders and swollen ankles are stuffed with organic waste matter, which is normally rejected through urine, sweat and bowels. Waste matter often collects in the connective tissue. Connective tissue is to be found in the body wherever there are no organs. Under the skin, it is known as subcutaneous cellular tissue.

In case of cellulite, the connective tissue fills with lymph containing much waste matter, which irritates it and causes it to contract. It then fills with water, which the body is prompt to supply in order to dilute the poisoned lymph and relieve the irritation of the tissues. If the process continues, the water thickens into mucus, which in turn becomes semi-solid matter. This congests the cellular tissue, which then becomes painful. This is cellulite. Cellulite is not exclusive to women; nearly 30% of cases affect men. Cellulite begins on the inside surface of the thighs and knees, covering up the bone projections. It quickly moves down to thicken the ankles. The thickness becomes more and more pronounced and soon affects the whole leg from ankle to the knee, over the mouth (the lower part of the face including neck) and thickening the lower limbs. The sides of the thighs swell out, the hips and buttocks become heavy with rolls of fat, the neck thickens and the shoulders become heavy. The cellulite has the following symptoms:

- The appearance of affected skin becomes badly nourished, rough, grayish and cold.
- Pinching the affected skin is painful.
- The affected area of skin gives a feeling of padding.
- Pinching causes bruising.
- The skin adheres to the underlying tissues instead of making for suppleness, becomes inflamed.

Neck, Shoulder and Chest Massage

Poor posture and round shoulders make chest muscles tense, Bad sitting posture, long drives, horse riding, sports, respiratory diseases (like asthma) put strain on these muscles. Massage can help stretch and relax the chest muscles, alleviates arching in the upper back and the neck and straighten the shoulders. Chest massage should be done before face massage and after the arm massage or stomach and back massage. For massaging the shoulders, lie on the back with a small cushion under the head, enabling the neck to be completely relaxed. Following movements are undertaken to complete the neck, shoulder and chest massage:

Stretch and Stroke Shoulders

Cup your hands round the shoulders, gently pushing them down together, then alternately. To stroke, apply oil, start massaging with hands below the collarbones at the base of the neck. Stroke the chest to the breast with smooth and firm pressure in case of women. Glide across the chest towards the shoulders. Swing your fingers round to the back of the shoulders and stroke towards collarbone. Knuckling, deep pressure, kneading and alternate stroking are some of the massage movements to release tension. The muscles of the neck are often taut and tense:

- **Alternate stroking:** Stroke with alternate hands on each side of the neck from shoulders to the base of the skull. You may use both hands to massage on one side of the neck from shoulder to the base of the skull. Repeat few times, then change the side of the neck.
- **Side stretch:** Cup the shoulder with one hand and place the other hand at the base of the skull on the same side. Push shoulders down and pull the head to stretch the neck smoothly. Now repeat on the other side.
- **Pressure stroking:** Put firm, circular pressure on both side of the spine with middle fingers of hands. Work up the neck and press into the hollow above the spine. Now press firmly at the base of the skull.
- **Pressure movement:** Stretch the neck smoothly avoiding jerking or pulling. Cup the hands at the base of the skull and give a gentle stretch to the neck two to three times. Now press the head between the cupped hands on the back of the head and over the

forehead gently. Move head up and down as well as on the sides, until the head moves freely.

The cellulite overweight doesn't bring the organic disorders caused by obesity. You can die from obesity — you will not die of cellulite. More serious cellulite will give rise to nervous pressure, resulting in severe pains, which becomes terrible if not looked timely. It is observed that a mother suffering from cellulite may have a cellulitic daughter. You can improve the look of your cellulite-laced hips, thighs and backside when you lose any extra fat through weight loss and exercise to tone muscles. Follow the exercises that tone your thighs, hips and lower buttocks — the areas prone to cellulite.

Overweight

If you are about 20% overweight, health risks soar for high blood pressure, cholesterol, diabetes, heart trouble and other diseases. Here are few simple tips to slim down forever:

- Physical activity is crucial for health and weight loss.
- You become overweight when you take in more calories than you burn up. Nothing burns up calories and fat like exercise.
- Walk for 15 minutes at lunch and another 15 minutes when you get home from work (if you are a working woman) or walk during evening hours.
- Exercise works faster if you also take a fewer calories. But do not have to crash diet.
- Chew the fat less. You do not have to leave out fat entirely, but you should keep it to 20% of your diet.
- Breakfast means break your nightly fast. Breakfast is the day's most important meal, because it's your body's signal that it's time to fight fat. While you sleep, your body stores food as fat. You are likely to lose weight if you start eating breakfast, even if you don't cut calories the rest of the day.
- Chew your food thoroughly and eat slowly.

- Water slows your appetite and keeps food moving quickly through your digestive tract. Drink a large glass of water ten minutes before meals.

How to Check Your Weight according to Your Height?

Height weight ratio (in inches)	Age ranges (years)				
	18-24	25-34	35-44	45-54	55-64
		For Women			
58	114	123	133	132	135+
59	118	126	136	136	138+
60	121	130	139	139	142+
61	124	133	141	143	145+
62	128	136	144	146	148+
63	131	139	146	150	151+
64	134	142	149	153	154+
65	137	146	151	157	157+
66	141	149	154	160	161+
67	144	154	156	164	164+
68	147	155	159	168	167+
		For Men			
130	139	146	148	147+	
63	135	145	149	154	151+
64	139	151	155	158	156+
65	143	155	159	163	160+
66	148	159	164	167	165+
67	152	164	169	171	170+
68	157	168	174	176	174+
69	162	173	178	180	178+
70	166	177	183	185	183+
71	171	182	188	190	187+
72	175	186	192	194	192+
73	180	191	197	198	197+
74	185	196	202	204	201+

- Low-fat desserts are deceptive. They are full of sugar and often contain as many or more calories as high-fat desserts. Excess sugar converts to fat when your body digests it. Instead, eat a piece of fresh fruit.
- Stay away from alcohol. Alcoholic beverages as well as alcohol-free drinks are very high in calories.

Underweight

Any unintentional weight loss of more than about five kilogram warrants medical attention. Slightly below average weight may lower your risk of heart disease, high cholesterol and diabetes. For women, the most important indicator that they are medically underweight is if they start having menstrual irregularities. This sometimes occurs in women who over-exercise or when estrogen levels drop when women don't eat enough to meet their needs. It is seen, underweight women who do not menstruate have a hard time becoming pregnant later. Here are few suggestions for underweight women:

- If your blood cholesterol is within normal limits, you can be less rigorous about fat. Try a liquid food supplement.
- Have a weight training program, preferably at a gym.

Diet Plan

Ask yourself to find out

- Are you really serious about losing weight? This will give you idea as to where the problem lies and how to solve it.
- How much do you want to lose weight? This will give an idea as to your approach.
- Within what period you want to lose weight? This will give an idea whether you want to go on a crash program or a planned weight reduction, which you can maintain long. Remember, what you have put on in ten years cannot be melted away in ten weeks.
- What method you wish to adopt to lose weight? You cannot lose weight by exercise if you have no control over the diet.

How to Know Your Ideal Weight?

Here is an easy way to calculate your ideal weight if you have average build. Take the standard as 56 kg for a height of 160 cm. For every additional height of 1 cm, add 0.7 kg to the standard weight and for every 1 cm less height, deduct 0.6 kg from the standard. 156 cm is a standard height for a common woman. A woman having 4 cm less height than the standard height of 160 cm will have to reduce 2.4 kg (4 cm × 0.6 kg). However, any weight between 52 to 54 kg would be normal for a height of 156 cm depending on overall body build and bony structure.

How Much Calories You Need?

An average woman would need about 1800 to 2000 calories a day. If one is of sedentary habits, the requirement of calories would be minimum for that age. If the daily activity involves great deal of physical exertion, or during phases of adolescence, pregnancy and lactation, the caloric requirement increases by a thousand calories. To remain healthy, well and agile one has to be conscious about the calories intake. A normal simple home-made meal (vegetarian or non-vegetarian) does not give more than 600 calories. However, one dish of 'kheer' or 'halwa' adds more than 350 calories. The daily pattern of eating should include at least two full meals, a breakfast and sugar-free fluid of beverages in between. If you have a tendency to overeat and gain weight easily, substitute high caloric foods by those, which are filling but have low caloric content, such as salads, soups, fruit and fruit juices, skimmed milk and thin butter milk. The best ways to expend more calories and burn up fats is to do brisk walking, jogging, swimming, cycling and climbing stairs. Balance the intake with expenditure of calories in your body.

How to Plan Your Diet Program?

Before you plan a diet, watch the following queries:

- What should be the right weight for age and height?
- If you are in the state of physical stress or suffering from any disease?

- How many calories you need in a day and its distribution?

Diet of a sedentary woman should include 1800 calories a day with the following ingredients (in grams):

Ingredients	Vegetarian	Non-vegetarian
Total Protein/day	60	70
Total Fat/day	60	60
Carbohydrates	255	245

A gram of Protein gives 4 calories, 1 gram of Fat gives 9 calories and 1 gram of Carbohydrate gives 4 calories. If you need more calories, add on Carbohydrates. Out of the total calories, 80% should come from Carbohydrates, 10% each from Fats and Proteins. This will produce less strain on your internal organs like liver, kidneys, heart etc. If you are a sedentary person, you need about 40 calories per kg body weight per day. An moderately active person will need 50 calories per kg body weight per day. In pregnancy and lactation, a woman needs about 500 to 1000 calories more in a day. An extremely active person busy in sports, aerobics, swimming, dancing can safely take 55 to 60 calories per kg per day to maintain a steady weight.

What to Eat and What to Avoid Eating?

Foods such as ghee, butter, deep fry items, syrupy sweets, pastries, puddings, aerated beverages, alcohol, red meat and fried fish give you plenty of calories. Whereas foods such as skimmed milk, watery fruits, fruit juices, leafy vegetables, dry chapattis and lean meat give you minimum calories. Foods like rice, wheat preparations, curries, lentils, pulses and underground vegetables provide moderate amount of calories. The body not only needs calories but also adequate vitamins and minerals.

Oils, fish, liver, butter, eggs, green leafy vegetables, coloured vegetables and fruits like mangoes, papaya, tomatoes, etc. are rich source of vitamins. Rice, maize, bajra, whole wheat, nuts and oil seeds, liver, kidney, dried pulses, yeast, lentils, dry peas, soya bean, meat, chicken, fish, cereals, oil seeds and nuts contain vitamin B complex (Thiamine — B1, Riboflavin, Niacin). Citrus fruits, goose berry (amla), mangoes are rich source of vitamin C. Plenty of vitamin D is available in fish, egg-yolk, liver, butter, ghee etc. and vitamin E in cotton seed oil, peanut oil, brown rice, whole egg, butter and coconut.

How to Fight Obesity?

- Burn up all calories that go in the body.
- Get your calories mainly from carbohydrates, not from fats and oils.
- Avoid intake of sweets and deep fried items in your diet.
- Avoid in between eating.
- Eat a bowl of salad or take a glass of skimmed milk before going to a dinner party.
- Put aside at least fifteen minutes daily not just for your bath but for toning up exercise as well.
- If you are hungry fill up your stomach with fruits, juices and butter milk.
- Do not skip a major meal-breakfast, lunch or dinner.

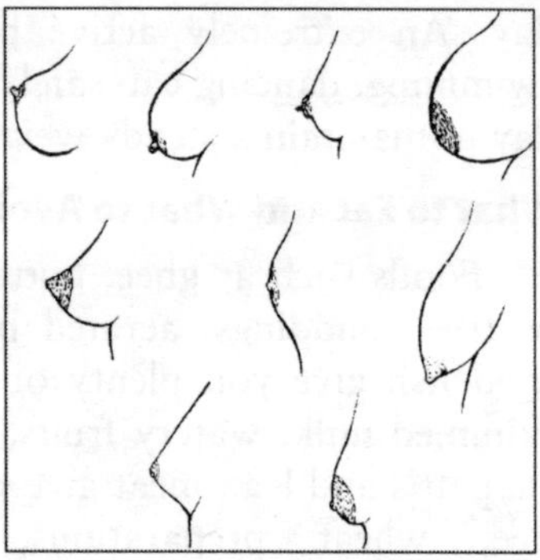

Breast Beauty

Women's breasts come in different shapes and sizes with different breast problems. Some women suffer from pain just before or during periods, others have the problem of swollen, lumpy, leakage of milk, under-developed or over-developed and saggy breasts. The mammary glands are composed of fat and glandular tissue. Due to adrenal and ovarian hormonal effects, the breasts begin to

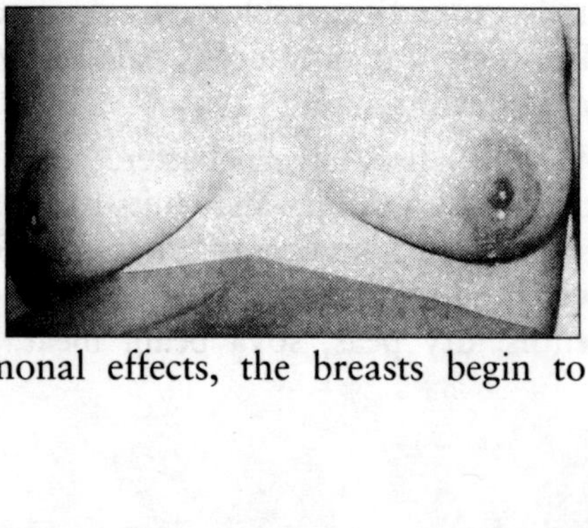

grow during adolescence and soon take the full adult size. There is another spurt of growth in pregnancy when glandular part of breast fully develops, and during this period the following care should be taken:

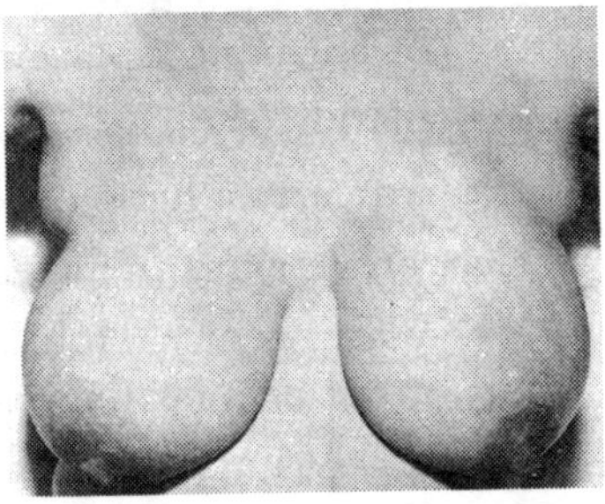

- The breasts should be supported by right fitting under clothes (bra).
- The skin of breasts should be kept clean to prevent boils, fungal infection and scabies.
- The nipples should not be handled unnecessarily. However, suckling of nipples is a good exercise of the breasts.
- Remember, the skin of areola and nipples is very sensitive to touch and sucking. If this part is dry and flaky, application of a little cream helps to smoothen the skin.
- A few hair stumps are always present even in the female breasts near the areola; never use depilatory cream or a tweezer to remove these hair roots.
- Breasts begin to sag with age, ill health, incorrect methods of lactation, poor posture, obesity and sudden weight loss. There is no get back formulae to get back firm rounded breasts except for plastic reconstructive surgery.
- The firmness or laxity of the breasts depends a lot on overall muscle tone of the body, constitutional tendency and exercises you make.

Doctors suggest a routine mammography (low dose X-ray of the breasts) once after every six months to detect disorders and cancer of breast. Mammography is a test to get clear picture of the breasts compressed between two plastic plates. The test is taken about one week after the last day of menstruation when breast swelling and tenderness is minimum.

A female should consult a doctor if she notices the following symptoms:

- Breast pain that comes on suddenly.
- Breast pain that occurs after starting new medication or hormone replacement therapy.
- Bloody or milky discharge from one or both nipples.
- Any breast lump or thickening.

Here are few tips to increase health and beauty of breasts:

- Warm gently. Hold a warm compress, such as heated towel or a heating pad against the breast for 10 to 15 minutes, which gives relief from breast tenderness.
- Cool down swelling of breast tissues which often occurs before and during menstruation. Wrap ice cubes in towel and mould around the breasts until the packs warm.
- Wear a correct size or a supporting bra. Sometimes, the weight of breasts themselves can contribute to breast pain or discomfort.
- Drain out excess milk from the breasts after feeding the child.
- Cut salt. Salt is a water magnet. If breast discomfort is associated with fluid retention, then reduce salt intake.
- Cut caffeine in all forms. Caffeine is included in coffee, tea, soda drinks, chocolates and pain-killing medications.
- Herbal tea available at herbal stores contributes to breast discomfort.
- Primrose oil tablets taken at night before going to bed relieve breast discomforts.
- Try some vitamin E, which is very effective in relieving breast tenderness and discomfort from fibro-cystic breasts.
- Eat less fat in your diet.

- Lose weight. Women store estrogen in body fat. Losing weight can help minimize the hormone's contribution to breast discomfort.

A good posture is an asset to every woman. If you are beautiful, you look more beautiful with an elegant posture. Posture is the way you sit, stand and carry yourself when you walk. But it has to be cultivated from a young age.

Broken Skin

Women and children prone to cuts and scrapes while doing household work, cutting fruit and vegetable, washing clothes and utensils and playing (by the children). Your skin is designed to repair itself provided care is taken to prevent infection and promote healing.

If the cut is deep to large—more than ½ inch long, you need stitches, which help the cut heal faster and reduce the chances of scarring. Any cut, which is deep enough to reveal a rich yellow colour has cut into the layer of the fat underneath skin and it must be stitched closed to heal properly. Apply pressure and ice to keep swelling down. You need a physician's care if:

- The cut area is red, tender, inflamed, oozing and discharge pus.
- You have fever or swollen lymph nods.
- You have multiple cuts and scrapes.
- The foreign material is imbedded in the cut.
- You have cut on your face or other prominent area on the body.
- You have artificial heart valve or a hip replacement.

A thorough repair is needed in the following ways:

- Apply pressure: Gently press a clean, damp towel against the cut or scrape for up to 20 times until the bleeding stops.
- Wash the wound to clean dirt out of the cut or scrape to avoid infection. Do not use hydrogen peroxide. Clean three times a day.

- Use ointments to dry. Moist wounds heal more quickly. There are several anti-microbial ointments available at the chemist shop to keep wound moist.
- Seal the wound with readymade bandage (called colloidal dressing) to fight bacteria and quicker healing.
- Leave the dressing on for a couple of days, it will naturally loosen and come off on its own or it will wash off in the shower.
- Protect the wound with a gauze bandage and tape. Apply the bandage loosely so that the wound can air out without being constricted.
- Change the dressing daily or two to three times a day.

Unwanted Hair on Face and Body

Unwanted hair, particularly on face is a matter of great concern, especially for women. There are several reasons for the growth of superfluous hair on the body, which include:

- Congenital causes.
- Imbalance of hormones, especially male/female sex hormones.
- Pregnancy and childbirth.
- Irregular menstruation.
- Mental tension.
- Long illness.
- Worries and shocks.
- Defects in uterus.

Immediately cure yourself of unwanted hair when they start growing instead of just feeling shy and embarrassed. On the face, superfluous hair grow mostly on the chin, above upper lip and on the forehead. Superfluous hair on the body, usually grow on the chest, arms, legs on and around genital area. In medical terminology, the unwanted growth of hair is called hirsutism. There are many ways to get rid of superfluous hair e.g. plucking, shaving, threading, waxing, bleaching and a permanent method Electrolysis — which was introduced by

Dr. Charles Michael in 1857 (the treatment acquired prominence in 1916). In this process, the hair roots are weakened by electric current. There are two methods in the electrolysis: the galvanic multiple needle method and the short wave method. The short wave method is much in vogue in India. The electrolysis should not be undertaken to remove hair in the following cases:

- Remove hair from eyelashes.
- Inner side of the nose and ears.
- From pimples or acnes.
- Being treated by a doctor for hormones deficiency.
- If suffering from diabetes.

Bikini-line Problems

Even if a woman has the figure and self-confidence wearing swimsuit with high-cut legs, there is always a problem of pubic hair. A depilatory (chemical hair remover) or shaving by the razor are not advised as the skin around the lower abdominal area adjoining the upper thigh is especially too sensitive and there is always a possibility of irritant reactions.

Mostly, women use razor for shaving the lower abdominal area to get rid of unwanted hair along the bikini line. This may end up with a nasty outbreak of little bumps and red rashes, which are the signs of a bikini-line infection. The skin in the bikini area harbors a lot of bacteria that a razor can pick up and drag into hair follicles—the pores from which the hair shaft grows. The infected follicles erupt into little bumps, a condition called folliculitis.

How to Remove Pubic Hair?

- Scrub the area before you shave. Scrub your bikini-line area with a antibacterial soap to reduce the amount of bacteria on the skin.
- Scrub again the whole bikini area with antibacterial soap after finishing shaving and rinsing off the shaving foam or gel.
- Pat the area dry with a clean, dry towel.

- Apply an astringent after you wash on the affected area.
- Dab on some cortisone and smooth it over the affected area according to package directions. It will soothe any irritation and help it heal.

Flabby Muscles and Saggy Skin

As we age, our skin loses elastin and collagen—the connective tissues that hold everything together. Elastin and collagen also keep skin flexible enough to stretch and contract the tissues at the time of pregnancy and weight gains. But when the body starts to produce less collagen and elastin, the skin starts to sag and the overall result is loose, flabby skin that just hangs. Weight loss is generally not the most effective way to beat flab under the arms, hips, thighs, abdomen and tummy. Weight loss can actually make underarms and several other portions of the body sag even worse. Women who want to get rid of extra flab especially under the arms by simple exercises and using light hand-held weights available at sporting goods stores.

Heavy Thighs

If your thighs are heavy, chances are that your mother's too—its the weight of heredity in most of the cases. If you want to get rid of the fat around the hips, you will need to reduce your overall body weight. Start getting most of your calories from low-fat or high-carbohydrate foods such as vegetables, chicken breasts, whole-grain and bread slices without butter. If you will lose weight all over your body, you will lose it in your thighs. The best way to burn off the fat is to get 20 to 40 minutes of aerobic exercise such as brisk walking, bicycling, step aerobics or running at least twice a week to increase your breathing and heart rate. Here are few tricks for creating the illusion of thinner thighs:

- Disguise it with dress. If your thighs are heavy, body-hugging knits, mini-dresses, skirts and flattering fabrics should be avoided.

- Wear solid navy blue or black skirts or dress having small patterns, which cover slim, thin thighs. Avoid wearing large patterns or horizontal stripes.

How to massage thighs?: Thigh massage relieves aching, stimulate circulation of blood and slim thighs. The following steps are advised for a perfect thigh massage:

- Stroke the whole leg from ankle to thigh with one hand on each leg, beginning at the foot, up the calf, over the knees and up to the top of the thigh, molding your hands to the shape of your leg and thigh.
- Knead the thigh rhythmically, squeezing and releasing the flesh. Now soothe from the knee with one hand following the other to improve shape and texture of the skin of your thighs.
- Pummel the thigh with loosely clenched fists of your hands, which bring blood to the surface and relieve stiffness in the nerves.
- Stroke your knees softly with circular pressure massage with your fingertips.
- Finally knead your calf muscles, squeeze with both hands, exerting the bone.

Saggy Breasts

With advancing age, breasts loose their attraction. Every woman has a desire to keep her breasts firm and youthful as long as possible. They add to your sex appeal. After the age of 40, breasts start drooping towards the waist. Besides being attractive, breasts are functional units of milk glands and fat supported by muscles of the chest. Unfortunately, over the time the ligaments from which breasts are suspended stretch and breasts start sagging.

Once a woman reach forties, the skin becomes more lax, the milk ducts shrink and fat replaces the ducts. This process tends to occur earlier in women who have had children and breastfed. Plastic surgery prevents breasts from sagging, but the treatment is very costly and painful. However, you can prevent your breasts from sagging and give them lift by the following methods:

- To build more muscles, try using a pair of weights. Pick up one weight in each hand when lie back on the floor. Extend arms out at shoulder level with your palms up clutching weights. The weights should be parallel to your body. Return to initial position and repeat the exercise 10 to 15 times. Gradually increase weight.
- Regular practice of *Bhujang yogic asana* (Cobra posture) proves very useful for saggy breasts. To practice this posture, lie on the floor on your stomach. Place your palms to the sides of the chest. Inhale. Raise your head and trunk slowly leaning back as far as possible without raising the abdominal region. Hold position for few seconds. Return to initial position exhaling slowly. Repeat this posture for three to four times. This asana helps to strengthen breast muscles, especially beneficial for over-developed or under-developed breasts.

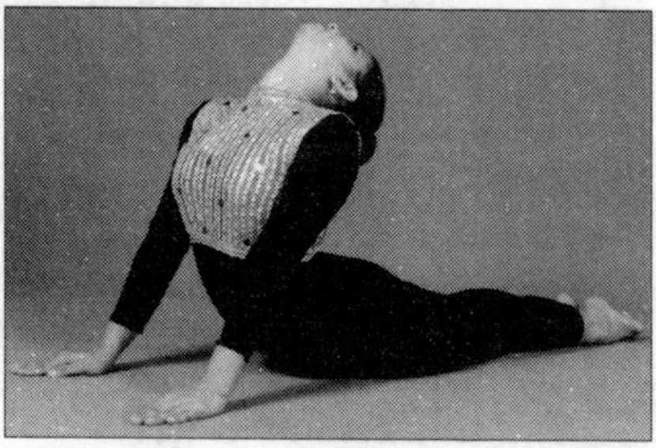

- *Dhanur Asana* (Bow Posture) is another yogic exercise for breast beauty to strengthen the muscles of breast and prevent fat from forming around them. To do this posture, lie on stomach as in case of *Bhujang Asana* and raise the legs along with upper part of the body and take the ankles in hands while arching the back.
- Don't forget sunscreen, since sun exposure can speed up the ageing of the elastin fibers that keep skin sagging. Make sure to wear a sunscreen whenever you wear a sundress or a bathing suit with a low neckline.
- Wear a bra.

Lines and Wrinkles on the Face

Doctors say that too much sun exposure causes wrinkles. About 95% of the sun's wrinkling rays hit the Earth between 11 a.m. to 3 p.m. Fine lines are shallow grooves in the epidermis, which can be made to look less obvious by the use of cosmetic products that improve hydration and suppleness. Wrinkles are of two types: permanent and non-permanent. Permanent wrinkles are present as a deep wrinkle on sun-exposed skin such as face and neck and do not disappear on stretching. The other type is a fine, shallow wrinkle that develops on the sun-protected skin such as abdomen and bottom, where the skin becomes thin and wrinkles easily as subcutaneous fat tissues decrease with age, and these wrinkles disappear easily on stretching. Cosmetic products cannot reverse wrinkle as the development wrinkles are the effect of changes in the dermis.

As we grow older, fine lines and wrinkles begin to develop. The skin loses its firmness and elasticity. Expression lines on the face and the patches of discolouration on areas of dilated blood vessels appear. The reasons for these changes are due to sluggish blood circulation and slow metabolism. Chemical changes take place in the tissues, sebaceous glands diminish in size and number, collagen production breaks down and hormone production is altered or reduced.

The Prominent Causes of Formation of Wrinkles

- **The effect of hormones:** There is a relationship between beauty and hormones. Lack or excess of hormones in human body or their imbalance can prove disastrous. Hormones are of various types, but the one associated with wrinkling and ageing are androgens, estrogens, thyroids, steroids, insulin and sex hormones. Androgens produced in the adrenal glands in women are basically male hormones. Excessive secretions of androgens activate the production of sebum causing acne or hair loss. Estrogens are normally female hormones produced by the ovaries, reduce secretion of sebum thus curing acne and pimples. The shortage of thyroid hormones secreted by thyroid glands makes the skin dry and wrinkled. Excessive production of steroids by adrenal glands cause skin infections, pigmentation and acne. The deficiency of insulin hormones harm complexion resulting in skin fungus, bacterial infection and itching. Male sex organs encourage growth of hair on the skin and body, whereas female sex hormones encourage growth of hair on the scalp.

- **Effect of smoking:** Avoid smoking to relieve wrinkles and ageing. Cigarette smoke and tar deprive the skin of the nutrients and oxygen it needs for good health, which leave the skin looking dull and lifeless. Cigarette smoke damages the skin, which lead to formation of harmful free radicals and weaken the collagen and elastin fibers resulting in the skin becomes permanently wrinkled.
- **Sun damage (Photo-ageing):** The prolonged exposure to ultraviolet (UV) radiation from the sun cause permanent skin ageing. Ultraviolet (UVA or UVB) radiation from sunlight accounts for about 90% of premature skin ageing. Both UVA and UVB rays cause damage leading to lower immunity against infection, premature ageing, skin disorders and skin cancer. A study reveals that people with fair skin when exposed to sunlight for just 5 to 15 minutes, metalloproteinases remain elevated for about a week. Avoid over exposure to skin, especially between 11 a.m. to 4 p.m. Ultraviolet intensity depends on the angle of the sun, not heat.
- **Rapid weight loss:** It can also cause skin to sag wrinkled by reducing the volume of fleshy cushion.
- **Use of lotions:** The fair skinned people should use tanning lotions readily available in market rather than fairness cream.

Sunburn Causes Wrinkles

While wrinkles on skin alone is not a life-threatening problem, it can be considered a form of scarring from the ravages of our environment, such as radiation and other toxins. The following precautions are taken in case of sunburn:

- Take aspirin or paracetamol to reduce inflammation and control pain (only with the consultation of a doctor).
- Cool, wet compresses or wear cool socks for 15-20 minutes four to five times a day, it will reduce body heat and control pain.
- Do not apply butter or heavy greasy ointment on the burned skin as these cause irritation.
- Fluid replenishment with an isotonic drink is recommended to compensate increased fluid loss through badly sunburned skin.
- Avoid sun exposure until the skin heals completely. As sun-damaged skin is more susceptible to subsequent burns.

Remedies to Reduce Wrinkles

The following natural ways help to reduce wrinkles and implant more youth in your skin:

- **Aromatherapy:** A facial mask can have a miraculous rejuvenating effect on wrinkles and ageing skin. Here is a self-made mask, which contains essential oils that help to stimulate the production of new skin cells and reduces fine lines and wrinkles. Mix the following ingredients in a bowl to make a paste:

1 teaspoon	Facial quality clay
1 teaspoon	Instant oatmeal or oat flour
½ tablespoon	Powdered milk
2 teaspoons	Honey
1 teaspoon	Avocado or olive oil
Sufficient quantity	Water
2 drops	Essential oil of frankinscense
2 drops	Essential oil of neroli, lavender or rose

Apply the paste in an even layer to clean face, avoiding eye area. Leave for 10 minutes. If it begins to dry before 10 minutes, mist it to keep it moist. Cover your eyes with eye pads moistened in rose water and follow with a cool water splash. Use this mask 2 to 4 times a month.

- **Massage:** Regular gentle massage helps to eradicate or reduce lines and wrinkles. There are several movements to massage different parts of the body (which have been described in the next tip). Use a massage oil containing four essential oils (2 drops each sandalwood oil, 1 drop each of geranium oil, lemon oil and cardamom oil) that nourish, soothe and energize the skin. Massage with your fingers gently using horizontal strokes.
- **Sun exposure:** The sun breaks down the collagen and elastin in your skin causing wrinkles. When you are out, wear a hat and a chemical-free sunscreen (made with titanium dioxide or zinc oxide), which has sun protection factor of 15 or higher. Then wash it off when you are not in the sun. Sunscreen is the best friend to clear wrinkles and offers protection from all the sun's potentially damaging wavelengths. Look for sunscreens that include oxybenzone, dioxybenzone, titanium dioxide, octocrylene—all that offer sun-protection factor. As an effective measure, apply it to the skin at least 30 minutes before going out as the ingredients need to be absorbed by the skin before they work. Reapply after swimming or heavy sweating.
- Don't smoke, since cigarette smoking deprives your skin of oxygen and nutrients, causing lines around the corners of the mouth and vertical lines on your upper lip.
- Choose cleansing lotions instead of soap. Soap foams up and makes skin feel squeaky, draws out natural oils from the skin and ages it prematurely.

- Limit coffee or alcohol. It can rob your body of water and nutrients and cause wrinkles on your skin.
- **Vitamin and minerals:** They are important to maintain youthful skin. Best food for the healthy skin is green leafy vegetables, carrots and fresh fruits.
- Exercise regularly.
- Egg mask helps cure wrinkles. Whisk an egg white until it's little frothy. Dab it with your fingertips or a cotton ball on your face. Let it dry. Do not move your face at all until egg pack dries. Rinse your face with cold water and apply moisturizer and light make-up. The egg white dries tight and shiny and tighten your skin to flatten out wrinkles.
- Tension leaves a harmful effect on the facial skin and results in the formation of premature wrinkles. Wrinkles, many times, are caused primarily by facial expressions, not ageing.
- Here is a youthful skin secret to relieve wrinkles. You may stay young with Vitamin E. Use Vitamin E oil or cream at night. Simply open a capsule of oil with a pin and rub it on the face

Stretch Marks on the Body

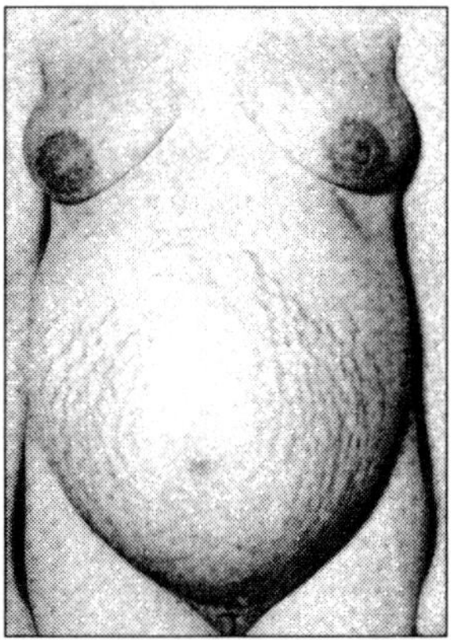

Pregnancy is one of the major cause of stretch marks on the body, the other is weight gain. Stretch marks occur on the breasts, hips, abdomen and stomach during pregnancy and other areas such as thighs when you gain weight. Stretch marks are triggered when skin is stretched to the maximum, which occurs when growth is so rapid that your skin's elastic fibers break. Stretch marks may cause by hormonal problems, certain diseases and medications. Remember, moisturizers, wrinkle creams and don't get rid of stretch marks, nor make-up covers them very well. However, vitamin creams work wonders. Exercise program helps to make stretch marks less apparent, but you should expect to see results in about two months.

- Start with 20 leg raises, which help to melt extra fatness from thighs, hips and abdomen. Lie down on the floor on your side, legs straight one on the top of the other. Now raise your top leg from the hip to toe as far as you can, then lower it back to the floor. Repeat 20 times.
- Do 20 inner thigh exercises: Lie down on the floor as above. But this time instead of raising your top leg, bend that knee and place your foot in front of your bottom leg and try to raise the bottom leg up about six inches. Lower the leg to the floor and repeat.
- In case of a pregnant woman who wishes to avoid stretch marks should from the moment you begin to show at about six to twelve weeks, apply vitamin C fluid to your abdomen every day. After the bath or shower, dry off, then put enough fluid in your hand to cover your hips and abdomen; rub your hands together and smooth the cream over your belly.
- Since extra weight create stretch marks, try to keep your weight on an even kneel. To control calories, avoid high-fat foods, watch your portions and get more physically active. Try to walk instead of drive, take the stairs instead of an lift or an elevator. Try to remain less dependent on your servant for domestic work.

10

Drugless Anti-ageing Therapies

There are many drugless rejuvenating therapies to control ageing. Various special herbal oils and herbs that trigger changes in the mind and organs of the body to bring balance and harmony to youthful system. These herbs and oils provide nutritional support, balance and youth to the body. Drugless therapies are credited with properties that help the body adapt to stress, achieve body balance, increase protein biosynthesis, elevate body enzymes, promote general endocrine synthesis, improve mental power, increase physical ability, fight free radicals and improve specific resistance to various stressors like heat, cold and wind. The following drugless rejuvenating therapies help to increase beauty of the body and enhance aging.

Shirodhara

Thin thread of warm oil is poured over the forehead and scalp. Shirodhara calms the mind, cleanses, balances the nervous system and relieves stress. Shirodhara is repeated three to four times a week for optimal benefits. Shirodhara is a deep relaxation technique that helps insomnia, depression, excessive mental or emotional stress and a meditative bliss. The treatment is followed by gentle head, neck and shoulder massage.

Shirobasti

In this technique, oil is kept on the head for about an hour in a leather cap. The patient sits on a comfortable chair wrapped in a blanket. Oil mixed to herbs is poured into the cap to cover hair/scalp. This treatment should be followed for 30 minutes to an hour depending upon the condition. Then gently massage head, neck and shoulder. Shirobasti is an exotic and ancient process to cure insomnia, chronic headaches, stress and anxiety, hair loss, premature graying of hair, improve skin complexion and premature ageing.

Nasaya

It is a procedure aimed at reducing waste products from the head, throat and body. Nasaya is the introduction of medicated substances into the nose, stimulates secretion, remove impurities of the head and neck. Nasaya treatment is used in headaches, nervousness, stiff neck, running eyes, ear infections, hair loss and to enhance facial beauty. This treatment can be repeated several times a week in conjunction with other therapies like reflexology and head massage.

Rasayanas

Rasayana means rejuvenate system. It is a beneficial treatment for the face and scalp to encompass a head to toe beauty along with other treatments such as massage (abhyanga), steam (svedna), use of herbs, pastes and masques (snehana), foot reflexology, aromatherapy, color therapy, gems and crystals, panchkarma (cleansing and strengthening) and kriya karma (rejuvenation). All these therapies and body treatments leave your skin looking and feeling fresh and young.

Siddha Massage

It promotes relaxation, calming of *Vatha, Kapha* and *Pittha*. It balances and increases the circulation to the body's largest organ: the skin. It also aids and facilitates the removal of waste products into circulation and removed from the body. Siddha massage increases lymph flow, strengthens the immune system and relieves muscle tension. This massage technique makes joints, ligaments and tendons mobile thereby adding to the flexibility of the body organs besides helping to calm, relax, tone and balance nervous system. It can be used to treat sleeplessness, regulate digestive and eliminative system, increase the production of collagen and elastin fibers and aid in the removal and preventing wrinkling an increase suppleness of the skin.

Abyanga

This treatment is recommended for muscle soreness, joint pain and stiffness, nervousness, tension, stress, restlessness, lack of energy, immune dysfunction, fatigue, tiredness, paralysis, poor digestion, poor elimination, sleeplessness and circulation of blood.

Lymphatic Drainage Therapy

This therapy needs gentle pressure on the lymphatic system to move waste materials out of the body quickly. This helps in controlling infections like acne, pimples and all problems of secreted skin type resulting in clear skin internally as well as externally. The waste materials are drained out through urine.

Seriatim Therapy

Constant mental tension leaves serious effect on premature ageing. This therapy is based on conversation between client and technician through touch and senses. By this therapy, emotions and mental activities of patient are controlled and he/she feels relaxed, and mental tensions get relieved.

Sandalwood Treatment

It is best suited for water retention, is diuretic and diaphoretic, leads to detoxification and stress-reduction. Cellulite triggers skin to sweat and release toxins, and acts as disinfectant. Sandalwood has been used for centuries in meditation and medicine. It creates spiritual cleansing as well as cleansing the physical body. Sandalwood unlocks trapped fluids and toxins been stored in the tissues and is a disinfectant and astringent.

Marine Therapy

This therapy helps in uplifting water level of skin in the body. In this therapy, various nodes and modes are uplifted by pumping technique and raising water level which helps in delaying ageing and fine lines, to control dehydration and improves lichen skin type.

Panchkarma: Means 5 Actions to Control Ageing

It is an ancient scientific system for detoxification and rejuvenates the whole system, bringing youthfulness. Traditionally, it is a preventive therapy aiming to cleanse all body systems by eliminating all the accumulated toxins from the body.

Panchkarma massage also known as a 'touch of health' relieves stress on muscles and internal organs. This therapeutic massage movement detoxifies the blockages inside the body and also beautifies the body giving a glow to the skin. Light and heavy movements, as well as vigorous and gentle rhythmic, soothing movements are given on different body organs to achieve beneficial results.

Spa Therapy

Spa therapy is used to treat problems like migraine, arthritis, spondylitis, paralysis, skin and hair disorders, diabetes, cardiac and vascular problems and psychological related problems like headaches, depression, fatigue, tension and mental stress etc. Spa therapy has been found to be very effective in curing not only various nervous and musculo-skeletal disorders but also help with relaxation and rejuvenation of body and mind to fight ageing.

Shiatsu Therapy

This therapy is also known as acupressure. It is used to treat disorders by pressing various pressure points on the skin of body. There are more than 500 Shiatsu points on the human body. Pressure on these points produce energy that flows in the body. To give treatment, the patient lies on the floor with face down. Keep both hands moving rhythmically along the meridians from one point to other pressing on each point from three to six seconds, which improves circulation and induce relaxation. To practice Shiatsu therapy, the following steps are performed:

- Press down on either side of the spine.
- Press down the buttocks and the back exerting light pressure on knees.
- Press on the points on the arms, hands and front of legs.
- Press gently in clockwise circles on points over the abdomen.
- Press on the sole of feet in line with big toe joint to energize the whole body.
- Press on one inch either side of the navel on abdomen to reduce fat accumulated in the belly area and energize the abdominal muscles.
- Press on the front about three inches below the navel to reduce weight, cure cellulite and improve circulation.
- Press in front four inches above the navel to energize the whole body.
- Press on the lower back, about one inch above the waistline at two points two inches away from vertebrae.
- Press on the lower back at waistline level on two points on either side of vertebrae.
- Press on the back working up on either side of the vertebrae towards shoulder blades.

Shiatsu Points on the Face

• Centre of hairline to the crown of head:	Relieves headache.
• On the centre of eyebrow:	Relieves headache and migraines.
• On the top edge of cheekbone:	Relieves headache and migraines.

• Grooves between the nose and upper lip:	Helps weight reduction.
• Between eyebrows:	Relieves headaches and migraines.
• Inside corners of eyes:	Relieves tired eyes.
• Below the end of eyebrows:	Relieves headaches and migraines.
• Small grooves at the side of nose:	Relieves facial tension, sinus, tooth-ache and clears nasal congestion.

Shiatsu Points on the Body (Rubbing)

• Grooves between the ribs:	Relieves chest problems and cough.
• Forearm muscle, at 2" below elbow crease:	Reduces nervousness and tired arms.
• Deltoid muscle:	Eases tension in shoulders.
• Outside the shinbone below knee:	Restores energy.
• Centre of abdomen around navel:	Cures constipation and menses.
• Skin between thumb and index finger:	Relieves toothache and ankle pain.
• Outer thighs below waistline:	Stimulates circulation in body.
• Crown on the head:	Relieves fatigue and headache.
• Base of skull above neck:	Relieves sinus and stiff neck.
• Muscles on the sides of spine:	Strengthens heart and lungs. Improves digestion. Strengthens reproductive organs.
• On the sacrum:	Relieves pain on lower back. Cures menstrual pain.

• Under the buttocks:	Relieves back pain and tired legs.
• Centre of crease at the back of knee:	Relieves menstrual disorders.
• Middle of calf muscles:	Cures back pain and tired legs.
• Outside or inside of ankles:	Relieves menstrual pain.
• On buttocks just behind hip joint:	Reduces tension in lower back.
• At the centre of palm:	Stimulates energy and relieves nervousness.
• Centre of shoulder blade:	Reduces stiffness in shoulders.

Aromatherapy

This therapy was started by the French chemist in 1926 to treat specific medical and psychiatric disorders with essential oils. Essential oils have a therapeutic effect on the body such as analgesic, antibiotic, anti-fungal, anti-inflammatory, antioxidant, antiseptic, anti-spasmodic, antiviral, carminative, depurative, digestive, diuretic, expectorant, hepatic, laxative, hypertensive and hypotensive, sedative, stimulant, toning and many more. The body absorbs essential oils through massage, which penetrate the skin and the lining of the lungs to be carried around the body in the blood.

Massaging the essential oils leave the following effects on human body:

- Restores balance to the emotions and mind.
- Soothes nervous tension and settle a worried mind.
- Improve concentration and memory.
- Calms anxiety and apprehension.
- Boosts morale and pacifies anger and frustration.
- Uplifts depression and negativity.
- Induces deep relaxation, relieving both physical and mental fatigue.

- Improves circulation to the muscles, thereby reducing inflammation and pain.
- Releases neck and shoulder tension and backache.
- Relieves neuralgic, arthritic and rheumatic conditions.
- Helps sprains, fractures, dislocations and heal readily.
- Promotes correct posture and improves mobility.
- Improves functioning of every internal organ.
- Improves digestion, assimilation, and reduces constipation.
- Stimulates the immune system.
- Reduces high blood pressure.
- Increases the ability of kidneys to function effectively to flush out toxins through urine.
- Flushes the lymphatic system by the mechanical elimination of harmful substances including toxins from bacteria and waste matter.
- Helps relieve headaches and migraines.
- Encourages deep breathing.

Detoxification: the Best Way to Remain Young

The present century lifestyle places high demands to look after the skin and fight premature ageing. To eliminate toxins, a regular deep cleansing of the skin is essential. You need a detoxification if:

- You are getting breakouts on the face, or on the back of the body.
- Your facial and body skin is too dry and looks chalky.
- You have dark shadows or circles around the eyes.
- Your skin looks gray and lifeless.
- You skin on upper arms looks bumpy.
- Your body feels no energy and you have a poor blood circulation.
- You suffer from cold hands and feet.
- You have cellulite.

How to give Your Body a Detoxification?

- **Giving massage:** It leaves a miraculous effect for improving the blood circulation and lymph drainage to banish cellulite.
- **Giving aroma treatment:** Mix 10 ml of carrier oil (preferably sweet almond oil) with five drops of a pure essential oil (lemon or juniper or grapefruit oil). Massage the skin of your hips, butt, thighs and abdomen as long as the blended oil is absorbed by the skin where applied. Massage only once a day.
- **Spa massage:** This helps in good blood circulation if applied after a bath, while the skin is still damp and warm.
- **Body brushing:** This is good for busting cellulite. Brush up your back, tummy, legs and arms towards the direction of your heart in circular, clockwise movement, preferably before taking bath in the morning.
- **Face masking:** It flushes out and helps to clear a congested skin using stimulating ingredients such as rosemary, eucalyptus and other herbs as directed by a naturopath. It has a re-hydrating effect on dry as well as oily skins. Apply pack for 10 to 15 minutes preferably before retiring to bed at night.
- **Epsom Salt Bath:** Having a bath with Epsom salt, preferably in a bathtub, helps your skin to eliminate toxins. Breath deeply while having bath for about 15 minutes.

Mud Therapy

Mud and clay packs are widely used since the ancient times as suggested by naturopaths. Mix mud and clay in equal quantity in warm water to make a paste. Apply the paste on the skin of your body, till it dries. Wash with water. The cool moisture in and under the pack relaxes the pores of the skin, draws the blood to the surface, relieves inner congestions and promotes heat radiations and elimination of morbid matter.

Mud bath of duration 30-45 minutes is found to tone up the skin by increasing the blood circulation and energizing the skin tissues. Regular mud bath improves the complexion, clears spots and patches on the skin.

Mud bandage, too, are beneficial treatments, when applied on different organs of the body as below:

- It strengthens the nerve system of the brain, cures headache, hypertension, mental tension and sleeplessness when applied on the head.
- It leaves beneficial effect on the psychic centre and fight anemia. It cures pregnancy disorders, frigidity among women and eradicate lines and wrinkles on lower abdomen after childbirth when mud bandage is applied on lower abdomen.
- In case of male impotency, the mud bandage is applied on male organ.
- For lung disorders, over-developed and under-developed breasts rub your breasts with dry towel to stimulate the blood circulation in muscles. Now apply mud bandage for not more than 15 minutes.
- Apply bandage on abdomen and waistline in case of kidney disorders, dysentery, uterus disorders, scanty and painful periods, irregular menses, all menstruation problems, profuse bleeding, leucorrhoea (white discharge laced with pus), spotting blood in urine, itching at the vaginal skin, vaginal odor and fatness around the waist.
- It has beneficial effect on weak eyesight, dark circles around the eyes, watery eyes, glaucoma and puffy eyes.
- It cures pus discharge, inflammation and ear pain, if mud pack is applied around the ears.

Ozone Therapy

Alkaline sprays are used on facial skin. Anti-allergic, antiseptic and sterilized powder is used in this therapy, which helps cure acne, pimples, spots and busts pussy infection.

Micro Therapy

This is a power massing therapy to treat ageing skin that shows signs of laughing lines, frown lines, crow's feet. This therapy helps to improve the blood circulation, stimulate nerves and muscles, regenerate cells and tissues, lift face, promote elastin fibers of the skin.

High Frequency Therapy

In this treatment, thermal heat is produced due to rapid vibration but without muscular contractions. The beneficial effects of this therapy include the following:

- Relieves dark circles and puffiness under the eyes.
- Rejuvenates crow's feet and shrunken eyes.

Derma Brasion Therapy

Various skin problems such as skin damaged due to acnes, facial scars, blemishes, tanning and pigmentation marks causing uneven skin tone are removed with the help of this therapy, in which the skin surface is leveled.

Anti-ageing Facial

It is a unique combination of powerful anti-oxidation and nourishing essential oils, which leave the skin velvety smooth and supple. This 50- minutes facial skin treatment is ideal for sensitive or environmentally stressed skin type.

Alpha Hydroxy Acid (AHA) Treatment

This facial treatment is recommended for fairness and all types of ageing skins. The following procedure is applied:

- Cleanse the skin with a cleansing cream or milk.
- Suction with the help of a softening milk.
- Apply alkaline scrub (optional).

- Steam the face for 3-5 minutes, followed by friction massage (or lymphatic massage) for 5-10 minutes with cream (mixture of skin food and gel).
- Remove blackheads, if visible.
- Tŏ remove infection, use high frequency and a protein mask if the skin is oily and prone to acne. If the skin is sensitive, apply whitening mask instead of protein mask
- Let the mask dry for 20-30 minutes, then wash off.

Hydrotherapy: a Technique to Remain Young till 100 Years

A healthy body is always beautiful. Hydrotherapy is a natural way of abating several body disorders. Water in various ways at varying temperatures in the form of pack or a bath is used. A hipbath leaves a relaxing effect, revives the dead skin, opens the skin pores, facilitates the escape of heat from the body and increases the body metabolism.

A hipbath is one of the most useful forms of hydrotherapy given in cold, hot, neutral and alternate temperatures. The treatment involves only the hips and the abdominal region below the navel in a special type of tub filled with water to cover the hips and reach up to the navel.

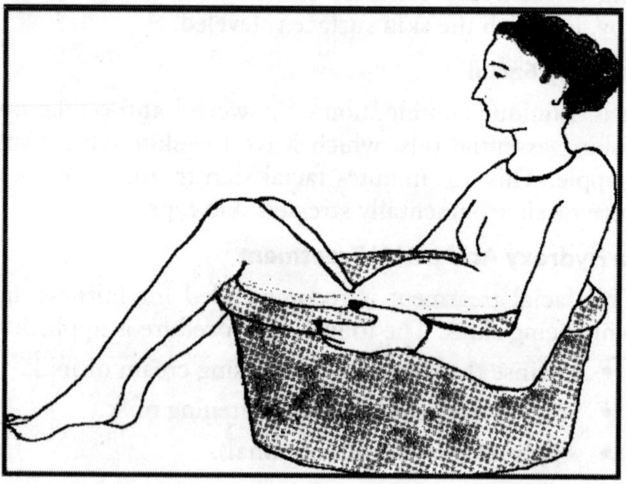

11

When Overweight Makes You Look Aged

Why Overweight?

Overeating is the sole cause for overweight. In other words, total caloric intake exceeds total caloric needs.

What's the Effect of Glandular Disorders on Overweight?

Glandular disorders have rare effect for overweight. Most of obese women seen overweight are usually over-eaters.

What is the Effect of Administering Thyroid Extract to Reduce Weight?

Thyroid glands control the metabolic rate and excessive dose may have a harmful effect and damaging the heart.

Should Injections be Given to Reduce Weight?

Doctors administer injections for reducing weight, which consist of diuretic drugs that leave temporary results, because they cause water loss in the body rather than decrease in fat tissue. There is no permanent weight loss due to such injections.

To what extent the Weight can be Reduced by Medication?

There are few medicines that cut the appetite temporarily to enable the patient to take less food but their result is not long lasting.

What are These Weight-reducing Drugs?

These drugs usually belong to the amphetamine group, such as Benzedrine, Dexedrine, etc. There are also certain cellulose products, which give the patient the sensation that stomach is full. In fact, such cellulose products are harmful.

What is the Effect of Physical Exercises for Weight loss?

Physical exercises play an important role for weight loss. However, short, irregular spurts of activity are ineffective.

What is the Best Way to Lose Weight?

To eat well balanced, medically approved low-caloric diet.

All Obese Person must Lose Weight?

Those suffering from ulcers or other intestinal upsets should lose weight gradually under close medical supervision.

What is the Hereditary Effect on Obesity?

A child born and brought up in a family of heavy eaters, usually become a big eater influenced by environments and tend to become obese.

There is no Weight Loss although Dieting for the Last over a year?

Such people do not diet carefully or at sufficiently low level of caloric intake. For desired result to reduce weight, adhere to a prescribed diet.

Will all Overweight People who Diet Properly Lose Weight?

They will lose weight, if their caloric intake is less than their caloric need.

What is the Relationship Between Life Span of a Person and Obesity?

Longevity is decreased in direct proportion to the degree of obesity.

What is Relationship Between Overweight and Coronary Heart Disease?

The evidence reveal that coronary heart disease is much higher among people who are obese and who eat high-fat diets.

What is Cholesterol?

A fatty substance found in certain foods and detected on chemical analyses of blood. The cholesterol level varies in different people.

What is Relationship between Incidence of Coronary Heart Disease and Blood Cholesterol?

Study reveals that those having higher ratio of blood cholesterol have tendency towards a greater incidence of coronary heart diseases.

What Type of Fatty Food a Woman should avoid?

Vegetable foods are not much harmful to increase blood cholesterol as compared to animal fats, which should be avoided as far as possible.

Are Massages, Baths and Standardized Weight Reducing Gadgets Help to Lose Weight?

They have no much affect upon weight loss of a person except psychological influence, unless they eat low-calorie diet.

Should People Dieting Strenuously take Vitamin Supplements?

If they are on an unbalanced weight-reducing diet, vitamin supplements are required. However, a weight-reducing well-balanced diet doesn't need additional vitamin supplements.

What is the Effect of Smoking on Weight Gain?

Smoking has a tendency to cut one's appetite. But usually those people who stop smoking are seen diverting towards sweets, fried foods and calorie increasing diets instead of cigarette smoking and start gaining weight.

Is There any Affect of Taking Alcoholic Beverages on Obesity?

An average glass of alcoholic drink contain about 100 calories and stimulate appetite.

Does Strenuous Dieting tend to Make one Nervous?

Only to those persons, who feel frustrated by eating less than their desire.

Weight-reducing Diets Cause Constipation?

Sometimes occur because the total mass of food intake reduces. Seek medical advice in order to aid bowel evacuation.

Should Children as well as Adults go on Low-calorie Diets to lose Weight?

It is very important for children to maintain normal required weight as poor eating habits among children make them obese not only in childhood, even when they are adult. Children can be made to gain weight by establishment of habits, which lessen food intake, such as:

- Avoiding excess physical activity.
- Avoiding emotional strain on them.
- Not to punish or threatening them.

Excess Weight-loss is Harmful?

It is.

Are those having excess weight more Prone to Develop Diabetes and Heart Diseases?

They are even tumours and cancer are more common among the obese than among the thin.

What is the Effect of Salt on Weight Loss?

Salt-restriction permits a greater loss of fluid and therefore has a greater weight loss. However, this is a temporary loss.

Is it Possible to Reduce Extra Weight only from Hips?

There is no efficient means for losing weight from a particular area of the anatomy. All such claims are baseless. However, exercises to stimulate muscles of the hips will help to reduce extra flesh on the hips.

What are common causes for Underweight?

- Chronic infections or diseases such as tuberculosis, kidney ailments, chronic liver disorders etc.
- Glandular imbalance such as excessive activity of thyroid glands or malfunctioning of the pituitary glands.

- Poor eating habits usually associated with an irregular life, excess physical activity and less sleep.

Does Emotional Strain Affects Weight and what's the best way to Gain Weight?

Usually people under emotional strain eat less, resulting in lose weight. Underweight people must eat more calories than they use. A thorough search must be carried out to make sure there is no infection or a physical cause for the underweight.

When the Weight Doesn't Increase Apart from Eating Large Quantity of Food, What would be the Cause? What is the best way to Gain Weight?

Eating too much low-caloric value food doesn't increase weight. Such people should be placed upon foods containing higher caloric value, such as cream, eggs, carbohydrates, butter etc. They may also burn up more energy with more-than-normal amount of sleep.

Following tips help to gain weight:

- Eat several full meals a day consisting of foods containing high-caloric value.
- Develop eating habits with four or five meals a day instead of three meals a day.
- Do not feel emotionally upset. Find out the psychological cause and attempt to eliminate it.

What are the Medications that can Aid One to Eat More?

There are stimulants to increase the appetite, but generally their affect is unsatisfactory.

Sudden Weight Gain or Loss

Your weight changes slightly from day to day even when you eat normal amounts of food. Dieting, as well as over-eating cause weight changes. But all changes do not come from gain or losses of fat. You might lose large quantity of fluid in a single day from sweating if you are doing hard labour. Changes in hormone levels during the menstrual cycle or eating a lot of salty food can make your body hold fluids and may cause to gain weight in a short time. Many medicines are available in the market, which cause loss of appetite and loss of weight resulting in depression. Weight gain or weight loss can be a sign of a hidden disease. If you gain or lose more than 7-8 kilos of weight in a month for no reason, you must immediately contact a doctor.

In case of a sudden weight gain with the following symptoms:

- Rapid weight gain with swelling in legs ankles and midriff.
- Fatigue
- Yellowed skin, bruising and bleeding.
- Impotence in males.
- Dark urine, black or bloody stools.
- Blood in vomit.

Causes may be the following:

- Cirrhosis (liver damage)
- Due to alcohol abuse.
- As a result of hepatitis or a disease passed on in your genes.

Consult a doctor for the treatment immediately.

In case of a sudden weight gain with the following symptoms:

- Swelling in legs, ankles and midriff.
- Shortness of breath and fatigue.
- Need to urinate often.
- Loss of appetite.

It may be due to:

- Congestive heart failure.
- A kidney disease.

If you have severe chest pain or shortness of breath, rush to a nearby hospital.

In case of slow weight gain with the following symptoms:

- Swollen face, fat on torso and upper back.
- Fatigue.
- Acne or a reddish skin.
- Trouble sleeping.

- Impotence or a breast growth in males.
- Unwanted hair on the face in females.
- Menstruation defects (stoppage of menses or irregular periods).

It may be due to the following reasons:

- Cushing's syndrome — adrenal glands make too much of a stress hormone that affects connective tissue.
- Caused by taking cortico-steroids for rheumatoid arthritis,
- Asthma or other illness.

See a doctor for consultation.

In case of slow weight gain accompanied by fatigue, a dry skin, goitre (swelling in neck) generally due to under-active thyroid gland, then call doctor for advice.

Sudden Weight loss due to:

- Symptoms such as rapid weight loss, fatigue, extreme thirst, frequent urination and infections in vagina in females. It may be due to diabetes. Seek advice of a doctor.
- Rapid weight loss despite increased appetite, anxiety, sweating, rapid heartbeat and swelling in the neck (goitre). It may be due to overactive thyroid glands. Call doctor for examination.
- When the weight loss is accompanied by fatigue, vomiting, diarrhea, darkened skin, hair loss, feeling cold and change of mood frequently such as confusion, aggression or a depression. The weight loss may be due to Addison's disease, adrenal glands making too little of hormones that control metabolism and responses to stress. Seek advice of a doctor.
- Slow weight loss accompanied by fever, night sweats, swollen lymph nodes, repeat infections, fatigue, diarrhea and sores. It may cause due to HIV infection or due to AIDS. Visit a doctor for thorough examination and tests.
- Weight loss with changes or humps in skin, abnormal bleeding, digestive problems, changes in bowel or

bladder habits. It may be due to a cancer or growth of cells. Consult a doctor.

- Weight loss accompanied by diarrhea, fatigue, gas and stomach pains and bulky, frothy, foul smelling stools. It may be due to mal absorption, when intestines fail to absorb nutrients from food. See a doctor.
- Extreme weight loss from not eating much. It is accompanied by disturbed menstrual periods, depression and sometimes vomiting.
- Generally eating disorder. Consult a doctor.

Caloric value of important food products in day-to-day life Product (100 gm.)

	Fibre	Carbohydrates Sugar	Starch	Fat Content
Milk (whole)		4.8		3.8
Milk (skimmed)		4.8		0.1
Butter				82.0
Cheese		0.1		33.5
Yoghurt		6.2		1.0
Egg (boiled)				10.9
Egg (fried)				19.5
Fruit cake	2.8	43.1	14.8	12.9
Rice (white cooked)	0.8		29.6	0.03
Pasta (white cooked)		25.2	0.3	
Bread (white)	2.7	1.8	47.9	1.7
Bread (brown)	5.1	1.9	42.9	2.2
Roast Chicken				

Disclaimer

This book is not intended to take the place of medical advice from a trained medical professional. Readers are advised to consult a physician or other qualified health professional regarding treatment of their medical problem. Neither the author or publisher takes any responsibility for any possible consequences from any treatment, action or application of medicine, herb or preparation to any person reading or following the information in this book.